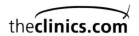

OTOLARYNGOLOGIC CLINICS

OF NORTH AMERICA

Congenital Anomalies of the Head and Neck

GUEST EDITOR
Glenn Isaacson, MD

February 2007 • Volume 40 • Number 1

SAUNDERS

An Imprint of Elsevier, Inc.
PHILADELPHIA   LONDON   TORONTO   MONTREAL   SYDNEY   TOKYO

W.B. SAUNDERS COMPANY
A Division of Elsevier Inc.

1600 John F. Kennedy Boulevard, Suite 1800, Philadelphia, PA 19103–2899

http://www.theclinics.com

OTOLARYNGOLOGIC CLINICS	Volume 40, Number 1
OF NORTH AMERICA	ISSN 0030–6665
February 2007	ISBN-13: 978-1-4160-4880-0
Editor: Joanne Husovski	ISBN-10: 1-4160-4880-4

The ideas and opinions expressed in *Otolaryngologic Clinics of North America* do not necessarily reflect those of the Publisher. The Publisher does not assume any responsibility for any injury and/or damage to persons or property arising out of or related to any use of the material contained in this periodical. The reader is advised to check the appropriate medical literature and the product information currently provided by the manufacturer of each drug to be administered to verify the dosage, the method and duration of administration, or contraindications. It is the responsibility of the treating physician or other health care professional, relying on independent experience and knowledge of the patient, to determine drug dosages and the best treatment for the patient. Mention of any product in this issue should not be construed as endorsement by the contributors, editors, or the Publisher of the product or manufacturers' claims.

Otolaryngologic Clinics of North America (ISSN 0030–6665) is published bimonthly by Elsevier Inc., 360 Park Avenue South, New York, NY 10010-1710. Months of issue are February, April, June, August, October, and December. Business and Editorial Offices: 1600 John F. Kennedy Blvd., Suite 1800, Philadelphia, PA 19103-2899. Customer Service Office: 6277 Sea Harbor Drive, Orlando, FL 32887-4800. Periodicals postage paid at New York, NY and additional mailing offices. Subscription price is $226.00 per year (US individuals), $400.00 per year (US institutions), $110.00 per year (US student/resident), $297.00 per year (Canadian individuals), $491.00 per year (Canadian institutions), $314.00 per year (international individuals), $491.00 per year (international institutions), $160.00 per year (international & Canadian student/resident). Foreign air speed delivery is included in all *Clinics'* subscription prices. All prices are subject to change without notice. **POSTMASTER:** Send address changes to *Otolaryngologic Clinics of North America*, Elsevier Periodicals Customer Service, 6277 Sea Harbor Drive, Orlando, FL 32887-4800. **Customer Service: 1-800-654-2452 (US). From outside the US, call 407-345-4000.**

Otolaryngologic Clinics of North America is also published in Spanish by McGraw-Hill Interamericana Editores S.A., P.O. Box 5-237, 06500 Mexico D.F., Mexico.

Otolaryngologic Clinics of North America is covered in *Index Medicus, Current Contents/Clinical Medicine, Excerpta Medica, BIOSIS, Science Citation Index*, and *ISI/BIOMED*.

Printed in the United States of America.

GUEST EDITOR

GLENN ISAACSON, MD, FACS, FAAP, Professor of Otolaryngology-Head & Neck Surgery and Pediatrics, Temple University School of Medicine, Temple University Children's Medical Center, Philadelphia, Pennsylvania

CONTRIBUTORS

OLGA ACHILDI, BA, Medical Student, Department of Surgery, Temple University School of Medicine, Philadelphia, Pennsylvania

STEPHANIE P. ACIERNO, MD, MPH, Clinical Research Fellow and Acting Instructor, Department of Surgery, Children's Hospital and Regional Medical Center, University of Washington School of Medicine, Seattle, Washington

SIDRAH M. AHMAD, BS, Department of Otolaryngology-Head & Neck Surgery, Temple University School of Medicine, Philadelphia, Pennsylvania

ONEIDA A. AROSARENA, MD, Assistant Professor, Department of Otolaryngology, Temple University School of Medicine, Philadelphia, Pennsylvania

VINCENT P. CALLANAN, MD, FRCS, Assistant Professor, Department of Otolaryngology-Head and Neck Surgery, Pediatric Otolaryngology, Temple University, Temple University Children's Medical Center, Philadelphia, Pennsylvania

HARSH GREWAL, MD, FACS, FAAP, Professor of Surgery and Pediatrics, Department of Surgery, Temple University School of Medicine; and Chief, Section of Pediatric Surgery, Department of Surgery, Temple University Children's Medical Center, Philadelphia, Pennsylvania

JASON R. GUERCIO, BS, Medical Student, University of Pennsylvania School of Medicine, Philadelphia, Pennsylvania

GLENN ISAACSON, MD, FACS, FAAP, Professor of Otolaryngology-Head & Neck Surgery and Pediatrics, Temple University School of Medicine, Temple University Children's Medical Center, Philadelphia, Pennsylvania

PAUL M. KANEV, MD, MS, Chief, Division of Neurosurgery, Baystate Medical Center, Springfield; and Clinical Professor, Department of Neurosurgery, Tuft's University School of Medicine, Boston, Massachusetts

PEGGY E. KELLEY, MD, Associate Professor, Department of Otolaryngology, University of Colorado Health Sciences Center; Department of Otolaryngology, The Children's Hospital, Denver, Colorado

MARGARET KENNA, MD, MPH, Associate Professor, Department of Otology and Laryngology, Harvard Medical School, Massachusetts Eye and Ear Infirmary; Associate in Otolaryngology, Department of Otolaryngology and Communication Disorders, Children's Hospital Boston, Boston, Massachusetts

LOIS J. MARTYN, MD, Clinical Associate Professor of Ophthalmology, Temple University School of Medicine, Temple University Children's Medical Center, Philadelphia, Pennsylvania

PHILIPPE MONNIER, MD, Department of Otorhinolaryngology, Centre Hospitalier Universitaire Vaudois, Lausanne, Switzerland

DARRYL T. MUELLER, MD, Post-Doctoral Fellow, Department of Otolaryngology-Head and Neck Surgery, Temple University School of Medicine, Philadelphia, Pennsylvania

TEJAS DINESH PARIKH, BS, Temple University School of Medicine, Philadelphia, Pennsylvania

KIMSEY RODRIGUEZ, MD, Assistant Clinical Professor, Department of Otolaryngology-Head and Neck Surgery, Tulane University School of Medicine, New Orleans, Louisiana

KISHORE SANDU, MD, Department of Otorhinolaryngology, Centre Hospitalier Universitaire Vaudois, Lausanne, Switzerland

MELISSA A. SCHOLES, MD, Otolaryngology Resident, Department of Otolaryngology, University of Colorado Health Sciences Center, Denver, Colorado

RAHUL K. SHAH, MD, Assistant Professor, Division of Otolaryngology, George Washington University School of Medicine, Children's National Medical Center, Washington, District of Columbia

AHMED M.S. SOLIMAN, MD, Department of Otolaryngology-Head & Neck Surgery, Temple University School of Medicine, Philadelphia, Pennsylvania

WASYL SZEREMETA, MD, Temple University School of Medicine, Philadelphia, Pennsylvania

JOHN H.T. WALDHAUSEN, MD, Professor of Surgery, Department of Surgery, Children's Hospital and Regional Medical Center, University of Washington School of Medicine, Seattle, Washington

JEFFREY S. WIDELITZ, MD, Temple University School of Medicine, Philadelphia, Pennsylvania

CONTENTS

physiologic and psychologic wellness of children who have these anomalies. Congenital nasal abnormalities may be overt or subtle and can occasionally cause life-threatening emergencies at birth. A discussion of nasal embryology and development provides the basis for the discussion of some of the important congenital abnormalities seen in clinical practice. The final portion of the article is devoted to several of the more common syndromes in which nasal abnormalities are encountered.

Congenital malformations may affect any part of the eye and the ocular adnexa. Developmental defects may occur in isolation or as part of a larger systemic malformation syndrome. Many malformations can severely impair vision, whereas others have only cosmetic significance, and still others cause no symptoms and may go undiscovered or may be noted incidentally on routine eye examination. Congenital anomalies have numerous causes, most commonly of developmental genetic origin. The genetic basis of congenital eye and orbit anomalies is just beginning to be delineated, and future research on the subject will undoubtedly broaden understanding of the developmental etiology, pathophysiology, and treatment of congenital ocular disorders.

Congenital malformations of the oral cavity may involve the lips, jaws, hard palate, floor of mouth, and anterior two thirds of the tongue. These malformations may be the product of errors in embryogenesis or the result of intrauterine events disturbing embryonic and fetal growth. This article begins with a review of the pertinent embryologic development of these structures. After reviewing the normal embryology, specific malformations are described. Recommended management follows the brief description of each malformation. An attempt is made to point out where these malformations deviate from normal development. Finally, management recommendations are based on traditional methods and recent advances described in the literature.

Congenital cervical anomalies are important to consider in the differential of head and neck masses in children and adults. These lesions can present as palpable cystic masses, infected masses, draining sinuses, or fistulae. Thyroglossal duct cysts are most common, followed by branchial cleft anomalies, dermoid cysts, and more rarely median cervical clefts. Other topics discussed include median ectopic thyroid, cervical teratomas, and branchiootorenal syndrome. Appropriate diagnosis and management of these lesions requires a complete understanding of their embryology and anatomy. Correct diagnosis, resolution of infectious issues before definitive therapy, and complete surgical excision are essential to prevent recurrence.

Congenital laryngeal anomalies are relatively rare. However, they may present with life-threatening respiratory problems in the newborn period. Associated problems with phonation and swallowing may prevent a baby from thriving. Stridor is the most common presenting symptom of congenital laryngeal abnormalities. Often, it is associated with dysphagia, aspiration, and failure to thrive. Endoscopy is essential for evaluation and diagnosis in most cases. The differential diagnosis includes laryngeal cysts, atresia and stenosis, vocal fold immobility, and subglottic hemangiomas. In this article, the authors discuss in detail the evaluation and treatment for each condition.

Congenital tracheal lesions are rare, but important, causes of morbidity in infants and children. Consequently, experience in their management is limited and dispersed. Given its small diameter, the juvenile trachea is obstructed easily by various natural causes, or following a surgical intervention. The diagnosis of a congenital, tracheal, obstructive anomaly is based on a high degree of suspicion in infants and children with respiratory distress accompanied by retraction. In this article, the authors discuss the various causes of these conditions, their diagnostic features, and the treatment possibilities.

Normal anatomy, embryology, and congenital anomalies of the esophagus are discussed in this article. The classification, epidemiology, embryology, diagnosis, and management, including outcome following repair of esophageal atresia with or without an associated tracheoesophageal fistula, are described. The diagnosis and management of less common anomalies, such as congenital esophageal stenosis and congenital esophageal duplication, are outlined.

FORTHCOMING ISSUES

April 2007
Facial Plastic Surgery: What's Going on in the Subspecialty?
J. Regan Thomas, MD, *Guest Editor*

June 2007
Neurotology
David S. Haynes, MD, *Guest Editor*

August 2007
Sleep Disorders
John D. Harwick, MD, *Guest Editor*

RECENT ISSUES

December 2006
Cholesteatoma
Christopher J. Danner, MD, *Guest Editor*

October 2006
Endoscopic Surgery of the Orbit and Lacrimal System
Raj Sindwani, MD, FACS, FRCS
and John J. Woog, MD, FACS, *Guest Editors*

August 2006
Revision Ear and Lateral Skull Base Surgery
Richard J. Wiet, MD, FACS,
and Robert A. Battista, MD, FACS, *Guest Editors*

The Clinics are now available online!

Access your subscription at
www.theclinics.com

Otolaryngol Clin N Am
40 (2007) xi–xii

OTOLARYNGOLOGIC
CLINICS
OF NORTH AMERICA

Preface

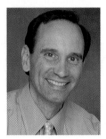

Glenn Isaacson, MD, FACS, FAAP
Guest Editor

Congenital malformations of the head and neck produce some of the most complex and interesting problems in surgery. Although major defects of the face and head may be obvious at birth, other significant abnormalities may elude detection until a skilled clinician identifies the telltale external signs of major internal derangements. How are these skills gained without devoting one's professional life to dysmorphology?

A basic knowledge of the key events in head and neck morphogenesis is essential. Embryology, which is a dry, sometimes painful subject in medical school, comes alive when used to explain the series of defects in a newborn. It is all the more important in planning surgical correction of these anomalies in a way that fixes the current problem and avoids creating new ones associated with growth and development.

This issue of the *Otolaryngologic Clinics of North America* has the goal of providing an intellectual and practical framework for dealing with congential malformations of the head and neck. Its authors come from several pediatric specialties and from medical centers around the United States and Europe. Each article reviews relevant anatomy and embryology, describes the more common congenital defects of the region, and touches on the medical and surgical treatment of these disorders.

We hope this volume will provide entrée into the world of head and neck dysmorphology for interested surgeons and pediatricians. Those who wish

doi:10.1016/j.otc.2006.11.014
oto.theclinics.com

to go beyond should consider three wonderful books by physician-scientists who have done so much in the past decades to advance the field:

Jones KL. Smith's recognizable patterns of human malformation. 6th edition. Philadelphia: Elsevier Saunders; 2006.
Gorlin RJ, Cohen MM Jr, Hennekam RCM. Syndromes of the head and neck. 4th edition. Oxford/New York: Oxford University Press; 2001.
Stevenson RE, Hall JG, Goodman RM. Human malformations and related anomalies. 2nd edition. Oxford/New York: Oxford University Press; 2006.

Glenn Isaacson, MD, FACS, FAAP
Department of Otolaryngology-Head and Neck Surgery
Temple University School of Medicine
3400 North Broad Street
Philadelphia, PA 19140-5199, USA

E-mail address: glenn@ent.temple.edu

ELSEVIER
SAUNDERS

Otolaryngol Clin N Am
40 (2007) 1–8

OTOLARYNGOLOGIC
CLINICS
OF NORTH AMERICA

An Approach to Congenital Malformations of the Head and Neck

Glenn Isaacson, MD, FACS, FAAP[a,b,*]

[a]Department of Otolaryngology–Head & Neck Surgery, Temple University
School of Medicine, 3400 North Broad Street, 1st Floor Kresge West, Philadelphia,
PA 19140-5199, USA
[b]Temple University Children's Medical Center, Philadelphia, PA, USA

Dysmorphology

Identifying a child as different or "funny looking" is a useful first step in the approach to anomalies of the head and neck. It is insufficient, however, to stop at this point. The field of dysmorphology has grown, in large part, from an appreciation that defects in development often have repeatable and identifiable patterns [1]. Knowledge of these patterns and an understanding of the developmental events that produce them have made medical genetics a science. Why bother to catalog such anomalies? As is the case with neoplasms or infectious diseases, if the clinician has "seen one of these before," he or she is more likely to arrive at an accurate diagnosis, to the search for other related defects, and to make useful statements about the future (Fig. 1).

Normality

What is normal? We accept a broad range of human variation within the definition of normal. Noses are big and small, straight and curved. By the same token, having no nose at all would be considered an anomaly by almost everyone [2]. Thus, defects in the head and neck can be separated into those that are gross malformations and those that are defects by degree (Fig. 2). It is important, therefore, to define the range of normal and to apply objective parameters to it. An example in the head–neck region is hypertelorism.

* Department of Otolaryngology–Head & Neck Surgery, Temple University School of Medicine, 3400 North Broad Street, 1st Floor Kresge West, Philadelphia, PA 19140-5199.
  E-mail address: glenn@ent.temple.edu

0030-6665/07/$ - see front matter © 2007 Elsevier Inc. All rights reserved.
doi:10.1016/j.otc.2006.10.012

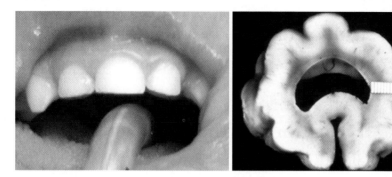

Fig. 1. A single maxillary incisor may be the only clue to a malformed brain in subtle forms of holoprosencephaly.

Measurements of intraorbital distance are cataloged, starting in the fetal period [3]. Measurements for an individual patient can be compared with these charts, and normality defined for any particular age group [4].

Normality of some other physical properties is more difficult to define. What is intelligence? How many colors should a normal adult perceive? What variations in the shape of the antihelix are acceptable? Students of human development strive to establish useful tests and norms for each of these important characteristics.

Patterns of anomalies

The clinical diagnosis of a malformation is rarely made on the basis of a single defect. Once one has identified a defect, it is important to know what other important or subtle defects might tend to occur in the same individual (Fig. 3). Some of this information comes from the collective experience of observers over the years, and some of it can be reasoned, if one

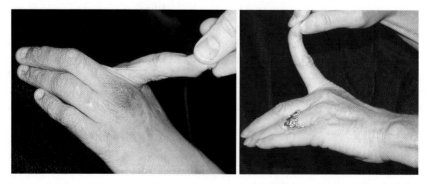

Fig. 2. How much joint laxity is too much? Ehlers-Danlos syndrome (*left*) versus normal digital extension (*right*).

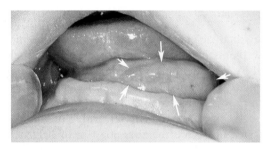

Fig. 3. This sublingual neurofibroma (*arrows*) was the presenting symptom in a child with neurofibromatosis-1.

appreciates the genetic and morphogenic processes that lead to the normal formation of individual features. Children with preauricular pits or tags are more likely to be deaf than children without such minor defects [5]. Starting with this basic information, a well-trained clinician knows to test hearing in any child with such a defect. More important, the dysmorphologist is aware of the existence of the branchio-oto-renal syndrome and recognizes that the development of the outer, middle, and inner ears are related (Fig. 4). Armed with such knowledge, he/she can look for the rest of the pattern and, finding it, make informed statements about the child's future and the probability that related family members or offspring will have the same disorder. Finally, awareness that ear and kidney anomalies occur together in a nonrandom fashion can lead the clinician to diagnose a hidden renal anomaly that might otherwise have been missed [6].

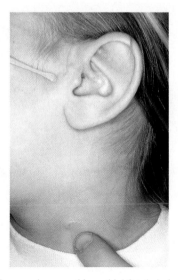

Fig. 4. Preauricular appendages and a second branchial fistula in branchio-oto-renal syndrome.

Variation in expression

For any individual defect, there may be variations in the phenotype, which can show themselves in a cohort or even in a single child. Within a family affected by Waardenburg syndrome, the presence and extent of individual features may be varied (Fig. 5). Although several family members with Waardenburg syndrome may have the same defect in their DNA, some can exhibit the typical broad nasal bridge of this disorder, whereas others lack this feature. One member may have heterochromatic irides, whereas another has clear blue eyes. One might be completely deaf, whereas another has only a partial hearing loss. Similarly, variation may exist within an individual. A genetic abnormality that causes malformations of a paired organ like the kidneys may affect only the left kidney and not the right [7].

Variation in cause

Similar morphologic features may arise from different causes. A cleft palate may be caused by a single heritable genetic defect [8]. A similar appearing palatal cleft may result from a growth abnormality in the fetal mandible that results in upward protrusion of the tongue and an inhibition of the midline effusion of the palatal shelves (Fig. 6). Yet another midline fusion defect might be produced by a benign tumor of the maxilla. Only by taking a complete family history, searching for associated anomalies, and looking for DNA variations can one hope to sort out multiple possible causes of a particular defect.

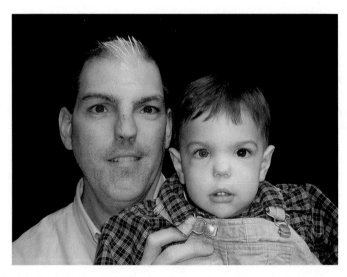

Fig. 5. A white forelock, broad nasal root and dystopia canthorum in the father, and heterochromatic irides in the son, affected by Waardenburg syndrome.

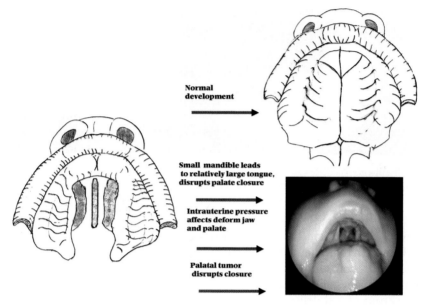

Normal
development

Small mandible leads
to relatively large tongue,
disrupts palate closure

Intrauterine pressure
affects deform jaw
and palate

Palatal tumor
disrupts closure

Fig. 6. Failed closure of the palatal shelves can lead to a broad U-shaped cleft. Several mechanisms can inhibit closure and lead to a similar defect.

Malformation versus deformation versus disruption

Most of the major defects identified in humans are the products of incorrect morphogenesis. Such defects, regardless of their cause, are described as malformations. Most of morphogenesis takes place during the first trimester of gestation. Some major defects, however, may result from pressure effects or other destructive phenomena occurring after the complete formation of the organism. Such events are characterized as deformations or disruptions, rather than malformations. In Potter sequence, oligohydramnios leads to poor lung development (which depends on the presence of adequate amniotic fluid) and flattening of the fetal face from uterine compressive effects late in gestation [9], which results in the deformation of an otherwise generally well formed fetus. In the amniotic rupture sequence [10], rupture of the amniotic membrane can produce constrictive bands that wrap around the fetal head or limbs, and result in infarction and disruption of otherwise well-formed tissue (Fig. 7).

Sequence versus syndromes versus association

Medical dictionaries continue to describe any collection of anomalies as a "syndrome." To the dysmorphologist, this term has a much more exact definition. A syndrome is defined as multiple defects in one or more tissues thought to be the result of a single cause. The classic example is trisomy 21

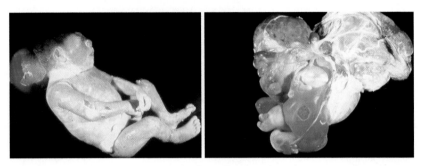

Fig. 7. An encephalocele can result from incomplete neural tube closure from folic acid deficiency (*left*) or from impaired calvarial closure in the amnion rupture sequence (*right*).

or Down syndrome [1], where a single identifiable defect (presence of a third copy of chromosome 21) leads to a series of anomalies (small stature, mental deficiency, hypotonia, flat facies, slanted palpebral fissures, small ears, cardiac defect, and so forth). Clearly, not all children with trisomy 21 have the same anomalies, illustrating the range and variability one can see with a similar chromosomal defect (Fig. 8) [11].

"Sequences" describe a series of defects occurring in a nonrandom fashion where a single event leads to a series of malformations. In the DiGeorge sequence, a primary defect in the formation of the third and fourth pharyngeal pouches leads to a predictable series of anomalies, including thymic

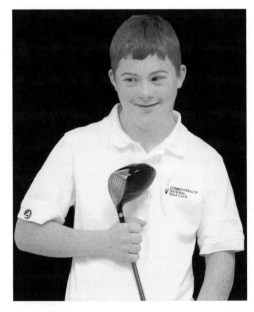

Fig. 8. John has three copies of chromosome 21. He is mainstreamed in school and plays a fine game of golf.

hypoplasia, absence of the parathyroids, and various cardiac defects. Although all these defects arise from a single inciting event, the underlying cause may be variable. DiGeorge sequence may be caused by prenatal exposure to alcohol [12], various chromosomal abnormalities (especially deletions of the long arm of chromosome 22) [13], or exposure to isotretinoin (Accutane) in utero [14].

The tendency of some malformations to occur together more commonly than would be expected by chance, yet not be part of an established malformation syndrom, is termed an "association." Such associations are often named as acronyms of their component defects. CHARGE association [15] is characterized by coloboma of the eye (especially of the iris and retina), heart anomaly, choanal atresia, retarded growth and development and/or central nervous system anomalies, and genital or ear anomalies (ranging from small ears without malformations, to major anomalies with sensory-neural or conductive hearing loss). Sometimes, with increasing medical knowledge, these loose associations come to be defined as syndromes or sequences. CHARGE was recategorized recently as a syndrome when mutations in the gene CDH7, a member of the chromodomain helicase DNA-binding gene family, were identified as its likely cause [16].

Much of the classic approach to dysmorphologist has been turned on its head in recent years. The completion of the Human Genome Project and the subsequent explosion in precisely identified mutations has confused the comfortable order morphogenesis. The paradigm, "gene leads to defect, which leads to syndrome," may not work well for all human malformations [17]. Gripp and colleagues [18] point out that two different point mutations may produce Crouzon syndrome (FGFR2, Cys278Phe). By the same token, the same point mutation (FGFR2) may produce either Crouzon's disease or Pfeiffer syndrome. Are these syndromes truly distinct? Why do these point mutations lead to significantly different phenotypes? It is possible that in the future syndromes will be defined by their molecular characteristics rather than their phenotypes? [19]. These and new, yet unimagined, questions are sure to challenge the field of dysmorphology in the coming years.

References

[1] Jones KL. Smith's recognizable patterns of human malformation. 6th edition. Philadelphia: Elsevier Saunders; 2006. p. 1–12.
[2] Hammond P, Hutton TJ, Allanson JE, et al. Discriminating power of localized three-dimensional facial morphology. Am J Hum Genet 2005;77(6):999–1010 [Epub 2005 Oct 26].
[3] Dollfus H, Verloes A. Dysmorphology and the orbital region: a practical clinical approach. Surv Ophthalmol 2004;49(6):547–61 [review].
[4] Levin AV. Congenital eye anomalies. Pediatr Clin North Am 2003;50(1):55–76.
[5] Fraser FC, Sproule JR, Halal F. Frequency of the branchio-oto-renal (BOR) syndrome in children with profound hearing loss. Am J Med Genet 1980;7(3):341–9.
[6] Kalatzis V, Sahly I, El-Amraoui A, et al. Eya1 expression in the developing ear and kidney: towards the understanding of the pathogenesis of branchio-oto-renal (BOR) syndrome. Dev Dyn 1998;213(4):486–99.

[7] Nayak CS, Isaacson G. Worldwide distribution of Waardenburg syndrome. Ann Otol Rhinol Laryngol 2003;112(9 Pt 1):817–20.

[8] Jakobsen LP, Knudsen MA, Lespinasse J, et al. The genetic basis of the Pierre Robin Sequence. Cleft Palate Craniofac J 2006;43(2):155–9.

[9] Scott RJ, Goodburn SF. Potter's syndrome in the second trimester–prenatal screening and pathological findings in 60 cases of oligohydramnios sequence. Prenat Diagn 1995;15(6): 519–25.

[10] Werler MM, Louik C, Mitchell AA. Epidemiologic analysis of maternal factors and amniotic band defects. Birth Defects Res A Clin Mol Teratol 2003;67(1):68–72.

[11] Roper RJ, Reeves RH. Understanding the basis for Down syndrome phenotypes. PLoS Genet 2006;2(3):e50.

[12] Cavdar AO. DiGeorge's syndrome and fetal alcohol syndrome. Am J Dis Child 1983;137(8): 806–7.

[13] Kelly RG, Jerome-Majewska LA, Papaioannou VE. The del22q11.2 candidate gene Tbx1 regulates branchiomeric myogenesis. Hum Mol Genet 2004;13(22):2829–40 [Epub 2004 Sep 22].

[14] Zhang L, Zhong T, Wang Y, et al. TBX1, a DiGeorge syndrome candidate gene, is inhibited by retinoic acid. Int J Dev Biol 2006;50(1):55–61.

[15] Stromland K, Sjogreen L, Johansson M, et al. CHARGE association in Sweden: malformations and functional deficits. Am J Med Genet A 2005;133(3):331–9.

[16] Lalani SR, Safiullah AM, Fernbach SD, et al. Spectrum of CHD7 mutations in 110 individuals with CHARGE syndrome and genotype-phenotype correlation. Am J Hum Genet 2006; 78(2):303–14 [Epub 2005 Dec 29].

[17] McKusick VA. The Gordon Wilson Lecture: the clinical legacy of Jonathan Hutchinson (1828–1913): syndromology and dysmorphology meet genomics. Trans Am Clin Climatol Assoc 2005;116:15–38.

[18] Gripp KW, Zackai EH, Cohen MM Jr. Clinical and molecular diagnosis should be consistent. Am J Med Genet A 2003;121(2):188–9.

[19] Biesecker LG. Lumping and splitting: molecular biology in the genetics clinic. Clin Genet 1998;53:3–7.

OTOLARYNGOLOGIC
CLINICS
OF NORTH AMERICA

Otolaryngol Clin N Am
40 (2007) 9–26

Congenital Malformations of the Skull and Meninges

Paul M. Kanev, MD, MS[a,b]

[a]Division of Neurosurgery, Baystate Medical Center, 759 Chestnut Street,
Springfield, MA 01199, USA
[b]Department of Neurosurgery, Tuft's University School of Medicine,
136 Harrison Avenue, Boston, MA 02111, USA

Congenital malformations of the skull and meninges occur as often as 1 in 10,000 births. Although meningoencephaloceles and craniosynostosis are apparent at birth, dermal sinus tracts may escape detection until much older ages. Arachnoid cysts are common incidental findings of neuroimaging of the sinuses or after trauma. The foundations of surgical repair of these malformations are based on their embryology and anatomy. Optimum management of children requires close cooperation between a pediatric neurosurgeon and multiple specialists involved with congenital defects. This article reviews the embryology, clinical presentation, and surgical management of these malformations.

Embryology

Beginning on gestational day 15, gastrulation initiates the complex tissue migration converting the primitive bilaminar embryo into three cell layers. The primitive streak begins as a thickening of the superficial ectoderm that deepens rostrally to form Hensen's node. Groove formation along the length of the primitive streak further deepens at Hensen's node to direct surface cell migration and interposition between the ectoderm and endoderm, forming the paraxial mesoderm. Further cell migration cephalad between the mantles of mesoderm, the endoderm below, and the ectoderm above forms the notochordal process. Extension of the notochord cephalad is limited by the prochordal plate and caudally by the cloacal membrane [1].

Division of Neurosurgery, Baystate Medical Center, 759 Chestnut Street, Springfield, MA 01199.
E-mail address: paul.kanev@bhs.org

0030-6665/07/$ - see front matter © 2007 Elsevier Inc. All rights reserved.
doi:10.1016/j.otc.2006.10.005

The notochord begins as a solid core of cells but cavitates from the primitive pit, forming the notochordal canal. During intercalation, the notochordal canal fuses with the ventral endoderm opening this canal into the yolk sac. On gestation day 17, the neurenteric canal (of Kovalevsky) penetrates from Hensen's node through the notochord communicating the amniotic cavity to the inner yolk sac. This transient channel is closed during excalation, with infolding of the notochordal plate in a cranial to caudal direction. The endoderm is reconstituted as a continuous cell layer, and the notochordal canal disappears. Mesoderm condenses about the true notochord, inducing formation of the neural plate and the vertebral bodies. With continued embryo growth, Hensen's node and the primitive streak are displaced caudally toward the sacrococcygeal region [2].

At stage XII of embryologic development, the cranial and cervical notochord separates from the adjacent neural tube, marking the site of the synchondrosis between the future sphenoid and occipital bones. Condensation of adjacent mesoderm eventually differentiates into the major bones of the skull base. Preliminary chondrification begins during stage XVI in the skull base and the body of the sphenoid bone. By stage XX, the hypoglossal nerve passes through a chondrified foramen, lateral to the foramen magnum. Vascularization of the cephalic neural tube begins at stages XII and XIII.

The bones of the calvarium originate from multiple ossification centers that surround the developing embryonic brain. Bone enlargement is induced by the expansion of brain volume and size. The development of sutures is initiated by approximation of the cranial bones. The sutures provide a dynamic mechanical union between adjacent skull bones, serving as the site of bone resorption and deposition. Fibrous desmocranium develops into an outer periosteum and an inner dural layer that fuses with the dura propria of mesoderm origin. Premature suture closure is often associated with anomalies of the cranial base. There is mixed evidence suggesting that skull base changes may be primary malformations or secondary to suture closure or both [3].

Flanked by mesoderm, the notochord induces growth of the neural plate and the vertebral bodies. The superficial ectoderm is destined to form brain, spinal cord, and skin, whereas endoderm matures into the gastrointestinal and respiratory tracts. The mesoderm guides maturation of bone marrow, connective tissue, skeletal muscle, and bone; a remnant of the notochord persists as the nucleus pulposis of the intervertebral disc.

During gestational days 18 through 27, the neural tube is formed by primary neurulation. Closure of the neural groove begins at the rostral neuropore in the region of the future hindbrain and continues toward the caudal neuropore. The anterior neuropore develops into the optic chiasm, septum pellucidum, lamina terminalis, and the rostrum of the corpus callosum. The posterior neuropore corresponds with the S2 level of the spinal cord. The superficial cutaneous ectoderm and neuroectoderm are rigidly adherent until neural tube closure has been completed. These layers separate during dysjunction, allowing dorsolateral mesoderm migration. The notochord and caudal end of the developing neural tube blend into a skin-covered, undifferentiated caudal cell mass.

Neuronal architecture develops about vacuoles within this primitive streak during secondary neurulation or canalization [4]. The vacuoles coalesce into a tubular structure that fuses with the more rostral neural tube. Regression within the caudal cell mass begins before canalization has been completed. There is condensation of the distal neural lumen, forming the cauda equina and filum terminale.

Meningeal development begins at stage XIV, and by stage XVI, there is a membranous roof surrounding the central cavity of the developing brain. During fetal development, arachnoid is the final of the meninges to differentiate. On rupture of the rhombic roof, cerebrospinal fluid (CSF) invaginates into the layers of the perimedullary mesh, stimulating differentiation between the subarachnoid and the subdural spaces. Pia matter evolves later from this inner mesh. This layer separation appears at a 180-mm crown-rump embryo length, at approximately 15 weeks' gestation. Incomplete separation of the mesh creates septations within the subarachnoid space. Dura develops from mesoderm cells of the sclerotome and develops continuous with the cells of the intervertberal discs. Dura circumferentially surrounds the developing brain and spinal cord by 80 mm crown-rump length.

Arachnoid cysts may develop when alterations of CSF flow lead to rupture of the primitive arachnoid septations. A diverticulum may invaginate, entrapping CSF in a noncirculating compartment. Another hypothesis is arachnoid splitting during delamination from the overlying dura. Arachnoid cysts may be associated with agenesis of the corpus callosum and anomalies of the dura venous sinuses.

The formation of dermal sinuses may reflect incomplete dysjunction [5]. Focal incomplete separation of the cutaneous ectoderm from the neural ectoderm during the fourth week of fetal development retains adherence of these layers [6]. Altered dysjunction can lead to the dermal sinus extension from the subcutaneous tissues to the intramedullary or subarachnoid space. Although the lumbosacral region is the most common location for dermal sinuses, they may occur anywhere along the developing nervous system, from the top of the intergluteal fold to the occiput or nasion. Disorder of notochord formation, with sagittal splitting of the spinal cord and hindbrain and persistence of dorsal cutaneoendomesenchymal fistula, has also been suggested as a alternative mechanism of dermal sinus formation [6].

The sinus tract is lined by columns of squamous epithelium encased by dermal and neuroglial tissue. Within the tract, nerve or ganglion cells, fat, cartilage, and fibrovascular meningeal remnants may be found [7]. Nearly 60% of dermal sinus tracts enter the subarachnoid space. Cranial dermal sinus tracts of the posterior skull frequently extend subtorcular into the posterior fossa, and intracranial cysts may grow to considerable size before diagnosis.

Dermoid and epidermoid tumors may arise within focal expansions along the tract in approximately half of all dermal sinuses [8]. These tumors are frequently encountered within the subarachnoid space, arising from congenital rests of cells derived from the caudal cell mass or mesoderm [9]. Dermoid histology is most common; epidermoids are seen in 13%, and teratoma and malignant transformations are unusual.

Incomplete mesoderm condensation into the space between the separating neural and surface ectoderm may contribute to encepahlocele formation. With limited development of the overlying cartilage and bone, neural tissue and the meninges protrude and migrate adjacent to the skin. Based on this hypothesis, the defects within the herniated neural tissue may be secondary changes. Other mechanisms for encephalocele formation include malformations of the anterior neuropore and altered ossification within the skull base. Several genes including sonic hedgehog may be linked with encephalocele formation.

Craniosynostosis

Premature suture closure occurs in approximately 1 in 40,000 births. Sagittal suture closure is most common (about 60%), followed by unilateral or bilateral craniosynostosis of the coronal suture (25%). Approximately 15% of children have trigonocephaly from premature metopic suture closure, whereas only 2% to 3% of cases involve closure of the lambdoid suture. Most craniosynostosis is sporadic; a history of suture anomalies is detected in only 8% of coronal craniosynostosis and 2% of sagittal X-linked suture closure. Hydrocephalus and intellectual impairment is rare in isolated single-suture craniosynostosis, in contrast to Apert's, Pfeiffer's, and other craniofacial syndromes.

There are many primary and secondary etiologies of craniosynostosis. These etiologies include teratogens such as aminopterin, dilantin, retinoic acid, and valproic acid. Other causes include shunted hydrocephalus, hyperthyroidism, rickets, and the mucopolysaccharidoses. Numerous chromosomal anomalies are linked with craniosynostosis [10]. When craniosynostosis accompanies a chromosomal anomaly, the phenotype of a craniofacial syndrome is always present. Autosomal dominant and recessive inheritance patterns have been identified.

Children who have dysmorphic craniofacial features and unusual skull shapes are typically referred for neurosurgical evaluation at very young ages. Premature fusion of the sagittal suture locks the biparietal skull dimension. Directed by the growth and expansion of the brain, there is compensatory growth of the adjacent coronal and lambdoid sutures, producing elongation and scaphocephaly. In a similar fashion, increased growth of the sagittal and coronal sutures adjacent to unilateral coronal craniosynostosis produces contralateral forehead asymmetry with brachycephaly. Expanding on Virchow's description of suture growth, Delashaw and colleagues [11], recognized the compensatory growth of adjacent sutures and bones, predicting the calvarium deformities encountered with craniosynostosis. Orbital dystocia and asymmetry is most common with unilateral and bilateral coronal suture closure. In severe cases of multiple-suture synostosis, there is insufficient orbital volume to accommodate the globe, and vision-threatening proptosis requires urgent surgical repair.

Since the American Academy of Pediatrics recommended the supine sleeping position for infants in the late 1980s, there has been an epidemic of occipital positional plagiocephaly. This acquired deformity has been estimated to occur in 5% to 10% of all children younger than 12 to 18 months. There is a parallelogram skull deformity, with contralateral occipital prominence and ipsilateral forehead asymmetry. The ipsilateral pinna is displaced anterior-inferior, in contrast to posterior-inferior displacement with true lambdoid synostosis. Whereas surgical reconstruction is warranted for correction of lambdoid synostosis, occipital plagiocephaly responds to repositioning, head rotation, and helmet orthoses [12].

Radiology of craniosynostosis

Suture anatomy is well defined by plain skull radiographs, which may be the sole imaging warranted for diagnosis and surgical planning of sagittal suture fusion [13]. Among a group of 85 children who had sagittal craniosynostosis reported by Boop and colleagues [14], there were unexpected intracranial findings on brain CT, including a benign tumor in 5%, prompting the investigators' recommendation for preoperative CT. In a recent review conducted by Agrawal and colleagues [13], the requirement for any imaging of isolated sagittal craniosynostosis was questioned. Three-dimensional (3-D) CT assists preoperative simulation of planned osteotomies and reconstruction (Fig. 1A, B). Postoperative 3-D CT imaging allows comparison

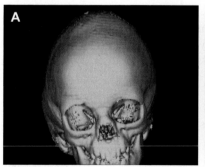
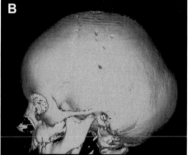

Fig. 1. (*A*) Anterior–posterior 3-D CT scan image of 14-month-old boy who had sagittal craniosynostosis. There is narrow biparietal skull dimension with temporal indentations. (*B*) Lateral 3-D CT scan of the same child showing elongation of the skull anterior-posterior dimension with occipital cup deformity.

with preoperative scans to assess the volumetric changes in the skull base and calvarium.

Surgery technique

Many techniques for craniofacial reconstruction have been developed. Dependent on brain growth for remodeling, linear strip craniectomy or synostectomy was the most common reconstruction technique for many years. Rapid bone regeneration was common, and caustic solutions or polyethylene applied to bone edges were modifications to restrict bone growth. The goals of contemporary reconstruction techniques are more extensive bone removal with active remodeling and reconstruction of the calvarium. Spiral osteotomies allow radical widening of the biparietal dimension in sagittal craniosynostosis and the posterior skull reconstruction in repair of lambdoid closure. The pi procedure was developed for immediate correction of the scaphocephalic head shape by active shortening of the elongated anterior-posterior skull dimension (Fig. 2A, B) [15]. Subtemporal decompression and barrel-stave osteotomies widen the biparietal dimension of the skull base. Repair of metopic and coronal suture craniosynostosis advances an orbital margin bandeau with forehead reconstruction.

Radical forehead advancement procedures were pioneered by Tessier and colleagues [16]. These techniques have benefited from the parallel advances in pediatric anesthesia. Rigid bone fixation is appropriate in the child older than 3 years; however, reconstruction in younger children must accommodate the final stages of brain growth and expansion, which is accomplished

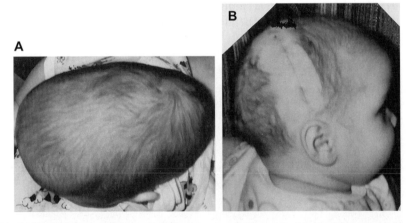

Fig. 2. (A) Preoperative photograph from the vertex of a 4-month-old girl who had sagittal craniosynostosis showing elongation of the anterior-posterior skull dimension with occipital cup deformity. (B) Lateral photograph of the same child, 3 weeks post posterior pi procedure. Following barrel-stave osteotomies for widening of the skull base, there was a 1.4-cm reduction of the anterior-posterior skull dimension.

with floating islands of bone sutured to the dura or the use of resorbable plate and screw fixation [17].

Minimally invasive endoscopic reconstruction techniques were first developed by Jiminez and Barone [18]. These techniques complete a wide-strip craniectomy of the involved suture through two small incisions. The endoscope provides sufficient exposure for the completion of barrel-stave osteotomies and craniectomy that extends to the skull base. Intraoperative blood loss and scalp swelling is minimized, and hospital length of stay is shortened. A dynamic cranial orthosis is necessary post surgery for nearly a year to maintain optimum head shape.

Irrespective of reconstruction technique, the risks of synostosis repair are low, with rare complications related to infection, blood transfusion, or orbital, dural, or cortical injury. Air embolism is very rare despite operative positions that frequently place the head above the heart [14]. Most synostosis surgery achieves an extraordinary transformation of the shape of the calvarium and skull base. Long-term follow-up is recommended to monitor skull growth, vision, and neurologic milestone development [19]. There is a small group of children requiring second-stage reconstruction.

Dermal sinus tracts

A midline cutaneous pit or dimple above the intergluteal crease is present in all children who have a dermal sinus. There may be associated cutaneous malformations including skin tags, lipomas, hemangiomas, meningocele manqué, or hairy patches. Hair is sometimes visible at the base of the dimple, and caseous drainage may be visible. The most common location of dermal sinus tracts is the lumbosacral region. Nasal, frontal, and subtorcular sinuses are encountered in fewer than 20% of cases. Family history of spinal malformation is unusual, and there is only a small male preponderance.

Dermal sinuses provide a portal for infection, and meningitis occurs in nearly half of all cases. The most common organisms are *Staphylococcus aureus* and *Escherichia coli*, followed by *Proteus* species and anaerobic organisms. Multiple organisms may be cultured in 20% of cases. Recurrent meningitis, despite successful antibiotic therapy, is common until the skin defect is diagnosed and repaired. The recovery and identification of organisms from lumbar puncture is more diagnostically accurate than culture of purulent material draining from the sinus ostium. Abscess formation may involve the epidural or subdural spaces, with extension over many vertebral levels [20]. Some children have repetitive sterile meningitis caused by contact of CSF with irritative dermoid or epidermoid tissue. Hydrocephalus may occur from scarring of arachnoid granulations from repetitive inflammation or low-grade infection.

Nearly all patients who have dermal sinuses have intact neurologic function at birth. Neural compression from inclusion tumors is more common with increasing patient age when the malformation has escaped detection during the first few years of life. Rapid neurologic deterioration suggests infection within subarachnoid dermoid tumors or from secondary hydrocephalus.

Radiology studies

Fine-section axial CT images with sagittal reconstructions following intrathecal contrast administration define boney landmarks and tract attachment to distal neural elements. Direct coronal CT is useful for visualizing anterior skull base stalk defects. Myelography must be avoided during superficial sinus infection because organisms may be introduced into the CSF space. Invasive contrast studies have largely been replaced by MRI, which visualizes stalk anatomy in three dimensions. Inclusion tumors are frequently isointense or slightly hyperintense on T1 sequencing and hyperintense on T2-weighted images. The imaging study of cervical dermal sinuses must include complete visualization of the brain and posterior fossa because tumors can be encountered within the fourth ventricle, cisterna magna, or cerebellar-pontine angle (Figs. 3A, B, and 4). If the sinus tract is above the skull base, then MRI of the brain demonstrates ventricle size and associated malformations. Gadolinium contrast-enhanced sequences can help identify the enhancement encountered with arachnoiditis, meningoencephalitis, or subdural empyema.

Surgical treatment

Cranial and spinal dermal sinuses should be surgically excised at the time of diagnosis in all patients, irrespective of patient. If the lesion is discovered

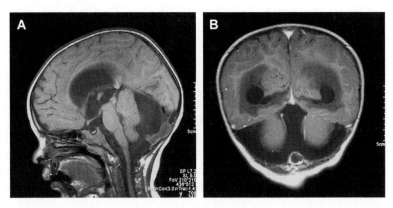

Fig. 3. (*A*) Sagittal T1 sequence MRI of a 14-month-old boy who had hydrocephalus and a retrocerebellar fluid collection. There is a subtorcular dermal sinus tract expanding into a large dermoid tumor mass within the posterior fossa. The dermoid tissue is slightly hypointense to the cortex. (*B*) Gadolinium contrast-enhanced coronal T1 sequence MRI of the same child. There is contrast enhancement of the borders of the dermoid mass and extreme hydrocephalus with transependymal CSF flow.

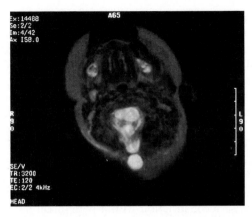

Fig. 4. Axial T1 sequence MRI of the cervical spine in a 6-month-old girl. There was a dermoid sinus tract extending from subcutaneous through the dura and densely adherent to the dorsal spinal cord. Ventral to the cord was an associated neurenteric cyst.

during an episode of meningitis, then exploration should follow sterilization of the CSF. Emergency surgery is required with rapid neurologic deterioration, recurrent infection during antibiotic therapy, or when infection cannot be quickly controlled.

An elliptic skin incision is made to fully excise the dermal sinus. Purulent material or drainage should be cultured in aerobic and anaerobic medium. The subcutaneous tissue is divided to expose the fascia defect, and the sinus stalk is circumferentially dissected. The stalk may pass between dysraphic lamina, across an interlaminar space, or through a full-thickness skull defect. The extradural path of the stalk may be variable, and surgical exposure must include wide access until the site of attachment to the dura is identified. The stalk of a cervical dermal sinus may extend through the foramen magnum and posterior fossa craniotomy, and exploration of the cisterna magna and fourth ventricle may be required (Fig. 5) [21].

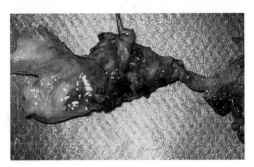

Fig. 5. Operative specimen of dermoid sinus tract with expanded dermoid tumor following resection from a 14-month-old boy. Hair strands are visible in the dermoid mass. Operative cultures from the tumor were positive for *E coli* and *S aureus*. The narrow stalk passed through a small subtorcular bone defect.

The dura is opened with an elliptic incision encompassing the tract. Intra-operative ultrasound is useful for identifying syringomyelia, syringobulbia, or intramedullary dermoid. Dermoid inclusion tumors are frequently multiple and can be solidly adherent to the spinal cord, cerebellum vermis, or within the fourth ventricle, especially when meningitis has occurred. Sharp microdis-section is necessary to divide adhesions, and every maneuver should be exer-cised to completely resect these tumors, especially if infection is present. Microsurgical confirmation of patency of the outlet foramen of the fourth ven-tricle is necessary during resection of posterior fossa dermoid cysts (Fig. 6).

During closure, the subarachnoid space should be irrigated with saline solution containing methylprednisolone, 1 g/L, to help minimize postopera-tive aseptic meningitis [21]. When the dura defect is small, it can be closed primarily, otherwise reconstruction with a pericranial patch is necessary.

Postoperative complications are limited following intradural exploration and complete resection of sinus tracts and cutaneous elements. Regardless of patient age, neurologic deficits or CSF leaks are rarely encountered. Men-ingitis or empyema clears with antibiotic management following resection of infected dermoid tumors. Long-term shunting is unusual for children who have communicating hydrocephalus following infection.

Meningoencephaloceles

Meningoencephaloceles occur in approximately 0.8 to 4 of every 100,000 births [22]. In North America, subtorcular and parietal malformations are most common (Fig. 7). There is a much higher incidence of encephaloceles in Southeast Asia, including Thailand, Malaysia, and the Philippines. In those regions, the malformations more commonly involve the anterior skull base. Nasofrontal and ethmoid encephaloceles may be large, with nasal and

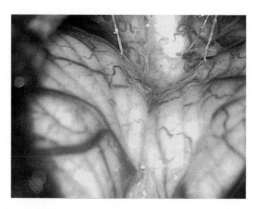

Fig. 6. Operative photograph of the cisterna magna in a 14-month-old child who had infected intracranial dermoid cyst and tumor. There were numerous arachnoid adhesions. Subdural em-pyema filled the cisterna magna, and the foramen of Monro was occluded by pus and caseous dermoid debris.

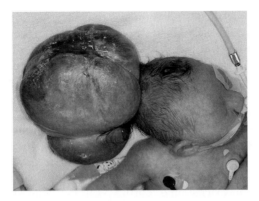

Fig. 7. Photograph of a large parietal encephalocele in a 2-day-old girl. The skin was intact over the dome of the malformation. There was only 1.5 cm³ of herniated cerebral tissue within the sac. The child did not have hydrocephalus.

orbital deformity with hypertelorism. Subtorcular encephalocele may be associated with other malformations including cervical neurenteric cysts and diastematomyelia. Herniated cerebellum and dysmorphic brain stem fills an occipital–cervical encepahlocele in the rare type III Chiari malformation [23]. Microcephaly and hydrocephalus accompany malformations in which there is extensive herniation of cerebral tissue and are associated with a higher incidence of seizures, developmental delays, and mental retardation. Chromosomal malformations are unusual, and family history of encepahlocele is rare.

Many encepahloceles are diagnosed in utero during transabdominal ultrasound or fast-sequence fetal MRI. Despite near-complete skin coverage, alpha fetoprotein and acetylcholinesterase levels in maternal serum and amniotic fluid may be elevated [24]. Prenatal diagnosis provides an opportunity for genetic and neurosurgery counseling and an opportunity for termination in severe cases. When the meningoencephalocele is large enough to challenge passage within the birth canal, elective cesarean section is recommended.

MRI is the preoperative imaging study of choice. There is ready 3-D demonstration of CSF within the malformation, extent of herniated cerebral tissue, and hydrocephalus. There may be associated intracranial malformations including agenesis of the corpus callosum and dysmorphic cerebral cortex. Magnetic resonance venogram (MRV) and coronal T1 image sequences are particularly useful for identification of dural venous sinuses adjacent to the malformation. Thin-section axial and coronal CT scans define the skull base or calvarium bone defect.

Surgery

The goals of encephalocele repair are drainage of the CSF within the malformation, reduction of cerebral tissue, and reconstruction of skin and dura.

When severe hydrocephalus accompanies the malformation, CSF diversion with a ventriculoperitoneal shunt is completed after encephalocele repair. Emergency closure is warranted when there is CSF leak, otherwise most repairs are completed in the first few days of life. To facilitate optimum reconstruction of nasal and orbital defects, the repair of nasofrontal and anterior skull base encephaloceles is usually delayed until several months of age.

The skin incision is made on the dome of the subtorcular or hemispheric malformation. Scalp flaps are elevated off the meningeal herniation until there is circumferential exposure of the bone defect. After entrance into the meningocele, CSF is drained and the extent of herniated cerebral tissue is identified. Small cortical tissue protrusions can be reduced intracranial. Subarachnoid hemorrhage and cortical venous congestion is common when there is a larger volume of cerebral tissue, especially following vaginal delivery. This cortex is frequently dysplastic with disordered cellular architecture and is generally resected flush to the dura margins. The dura is closed in a watertight fashion, and skin edges trimmed for linear closure. The dura and adjacent periosteum are osteogenic, and small to medium-sized defects close spontaneously with bone regeneration. Larger, persistent defects require delayed cranioplasty.

Encephaloceles of the anterior skull base and nasofrontal region are approached through a bicoronal skin incision. An orbitofrontal craniotomy exposes the malformation, olfactory nerves, and orbital margins. The extent of the herniated cerebral tissue or nasal glioma is best identified intradural. Dura repair can be achieved extradural or intradural. The reconstruction of the nose and orbits involves coordination and teamwork with a craniofacial plastic or otolaryngology surgeon. Bone graft is harvested from the adjacent calvarium.

Children are followed long-term in multidisciplinary clinics by specialists in birth defects. Serial imaging for surveillance monitoring of the ventricle size is performed, and regular developmental milestone and epilepsy assessments are completed. Poor neurologic outcome may be predicted by microcephaly, the presence of hydrocephalus, agenesis of the corpus callosum, and the volume of cerebral tissue within the malformation [25].

Arachnoid cysts

The population incidence of arachnoid cysts is low; autopsy estimates range from 0.10% to 0.7%. Arachnoid cysts account for about 1% of intracranial mass lesions [26]. Parsch and colleagues [27] reviewed 11,847 cranial MRIs completed at their institution between 1988 and 1994. Previously untreated arachnoid cysts were demonstrated in 89 patients (0.75%). Many cysts are incidental findings detected during diagnostic neuroimaging of the sinuses or following head injury. With the increasing use of prenatal ultrasound and the widespread availability of CT and MRI, cysts are being detected at an even earlier age.

The natural history of arachnoid cysts has not been well characterized. Most cysts are dormant fluid compartments that remain static during many years of serial neuroimaging. Only a small percentage of cysts progressively enlarge, exerting increasing mass effect on adjacent neural structures. Cysts rarely involute and disappear over time [28]. Arachnoid cysts can rupture after seemingly mild trauma, producing subdural hygroma and raised intracranial hypertension. Most arachnoid cysts are recognized during the first 2 decades of life, and nearly three fourths become symptomatic in children. The overall male-to-female predominance exceeds 2:1.

These cysts may develop anywhere within the subarachnoid space. In patients of all ages, nearly half of cysts occur within the sylvian fissure [29,30], and supratentorial cysts far outnumber those below the tentorium (Fig. 8). Less common sites include the interhemispheric fissure (Fig. 9) and the clival region. Cysts of the suprasellar region are encountered more commonly in children than in adults.

The optimal clinical management of arachnoid cysts remains controversial. Conservative management with serial neuroimaging studies is warranted in patients who have asymptomatic cysts. Surgical treatment is recommended in patients of any age who have focal neurologic signs or symptoms of elevated intracranial pressure. Intervention is warranted in children who have head size enlargement and should be considered in patients who have related seizure disorders. The goal of surgical treatment is the reduction of the pressure exerted by the arachnoid cysts on adjacent brain structures. The techniques for cyst surgery include craniotomy and cyst wall excision, shunting of cystic fluid to the peritoneal cavity, and more recently, endoscopic fenestration of cysts to the subarachnoid space

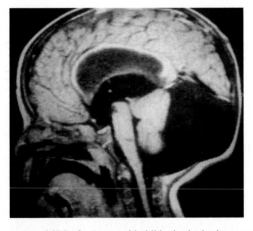

Fig. 8. Sagittal T1 sequence MRI of a 1-year-old child who had a large retrocerebellar arachnoid cyst. The cerebellar vermis was compressed, contributing to acqueduct narrowing and hydrocephalus.

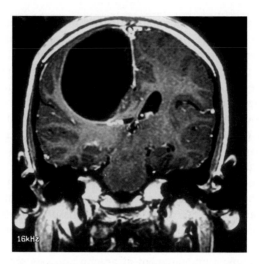

Fig. 9. Gadolinium-enhanced T1 sequence coronal MRI of a 6-year-old boy who had a convexity parasagittal arachnoid cyst. There is considerable mass effect on the cortex with subfalcine herniation.

or the ventricles. No single surgical technique has proved universally successful in the management of arachnoid cysts. Each procedure offers distinct advantages and limitations.

The advantages of cyst-peritoneal shunt placement include the relative simplicity and low morbidity associated with fluid diversion. Disadvantages include the numerous complications of CSF shunts, including infection, overdrainage, hindbrain herniation, low-pressure headache syndromes, and shunt failure. During microsurgical craniotomy, dense adherence of an arachnoid cyst to cortical and vascular structures may limit complete excision of the walls. With the recent advances in endoscopic equipment and surgical technique, minimally invasive fenestration is likely to become the treatment of choice [31].

Neuroimaging

Conventional radiographs of the skull may demonstrate deformity and thinning of the skull overlying an arachnoid cyst. There may be expansion of the middle cranial fossa or elevation and displacement of the sphenoid bone. Ultrasound through the open fontanelle of the young infant readily demonstrates arachnoid cysts and hydrocephalus. As early as 26 weeks' gestation, cysts have been visualized during prenatal ultrasound.

Arachnoid cysts are smooth-bordered fluid-filled lesions on CT. Cyst fluid attenuation is nearly identical to CSF, and the walls do not enhance after intravenous contrast. Deformity and thinning of the calvarium or skull base are demonstrated by bone window algorithm images. CT following intrathecal contrast demonstrates isolation or communication with the subarachnoid space.

MRI has become the preferred imaging study for arachnoid cysts. The extra-axial location of cysts and the relationship to adjacent neural and vascular structures are best demonstrated by T1-weighted sequences and magnetic resonance anteriogram (MRA). Cyst fluid is nearly identical to CSF on all image sequences, allowing arachnoid cysts to be differentiated from other cystic lesions including tumors and dermoid, ependymal, or epidermoid cysts. MRI readily demonstrates associated intracranial malformations such as agenesis of the corpus callosum, holoprosencephaly, or schizencephaly.

Three subgroups of sylvian fissure cysts were identified by Galassi and colleagues [32,33]. Type I cysts are lenticular collections at the temporal tip with little remodeling of the middle fossa. These cysts freely communicate with CSF in the subarachnoid space. Type II cysts are larger quadrilateral cysts, exerting moderate mass effect on adjacent neural and osseous structures. Type III cysts are large rounded collections causing severe compression of the operculum and insular cortices and midline shift with distortion of the lateral ventricles.

Supratentorial arachnoid cysts

Nearly one half of all arachnoid cysts in adults and about one third in children are located in the sylvian fissure. The most common symptoms are unilateral headache, typically in the supraorbital and temporal region. Seizure syndromes are the next most frequent symptom and may occur in up to one fourth of patients. The cause of seizures in patients who have arachnoid cysts is unknown but may be linked to compression of the cerebral cortex, cortical dysplasia, or subpial gliosis. Other symptoms may include proptosis, atypical facial pain, mild contralateral hand weakness, or hemiparesis. Large sylvian fissure cysts lead to macrocrania and suture splitting in young children.

Nearly 50% of suprsellar arachnoid cysts are diagnosed in children younger than 5 years and almost 20% present in children younger than 1 year. The most common symptoms include hydrocephalus, vision impairment, and endocrinologic dysfunction. Focal neurologic signs including gait ataxia, and opistothonus may be encountered when large cysts elevate and displace the midbrain. Male-to-female predominance is 2:1. Hydrocephalus develops in infancy when the cyst balloons superior, elevating the third ventricle and the foramen of Monro.

Type I sylvian fissure cysts are asymptomatic collections and require no surgical intervention. Conservative management is recommended with yearly MRI for 1 to 2 years. Adults and children who have symptomatic type III sylvian fissure or suprasellar cysts exerting significant mass effect require surgical intervention. Surgery is recommended for type II cysts when clinical symptoms are severe and out of proportion to the cyst volume.

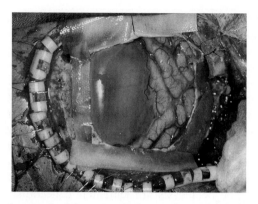

Fig. 10. Operative photograph of the parasagittal convexity arachnoid cyst seen in Fig. 9. The superficial walls of the cyst were resected and the mesial walls fenestrated into the interhemispheric fissure. Because of extreme thinning of the overlying dura, pericranium grafting augmented closure.

Craniotomy overlying the cyst allows excision of the lateral cyst walls and fenestration of the cyst into the basal cisterns (Fig. 10). Limited bone exposure may be assisted with frameless stereotaxic localization. After dura opening, the lateral cyst wall readily separates from the cortex, exposing the insula and branches of the middle cerebral artery. The operative microscope allows visualization of the tentorium, vessels of the circle of Willis, and the cranial nerves at the skull base. Multiple fenestrations between the deep cyst wall and the basal cisterns are opened with microsurgical technique.

Minimally invasive endoscopic fenestration of cyst walls is facilitated with frameless stereotaxic burr hole localization. The endoscope enters a sylvian fissure cyst tangentially, and the outer membrane is coagulated. Multiple fenestrations of the medial cyst wall into the basilar cisterns are opened with a Bugbee wire or with a balloon catheter. The medial cyst wall may be thick and resistant to endoscopic fenestration. Excess membrane manipulation may lead to traction injury on the adjacent oculomotor and optic cranial nerves.

When hydrocephalus accompanies a suprasellar arachnoid cyst, the endoscope enters the dilated ventricle from a frontal trajectory. After navigation through the elevated foramen of Monro, a third ventriculostomy and multiple cyst wall fenestrations are complete [31]. Following craniotomy or endoscopic fenestration, patients have rapid relief of headaches; however, the postoperative CT or MRI scan may not demonstrate significant reexpansion of the displaced cortex.

Summary

The surgery and management of children who have these congenital malformations require multidisciplinary care and long-term follow-up by multiple specialists in birth defects. The high definition of 3-D CT or MRI allows precise surgery planning of reconstruction and management of associated malformations. The challenging procedures of reconstruction of meningoencephaloceles and craniosynostosis can transform a child's appearance. For the pediatric neurosurgeon, there is little more rewarding than these outcomes.

References

[1] Lemire RJ, Loeser JD, Leech RW, et al. Normal and abnormal development of the human nervous system. New York: Harper and Row; 1975. p. 1–421.

[2] Pang D, Dias M, Ahab-Barmada M. Split cord malformation: part I: a unified theory of embryogenesis for double spinal cord malformations. J Neurosurg 1992;31:451–80.

[3] Hoyte D. The cranial base in normal and abnormal skull growth. Neurosurg Clin N Am 1991;2:515–37.

[4] McLone DG. Embryonic deformation and caudal suppression. In: Marlin AE, editor. Concepts in pediatric neurosurgery, vol. 7. Basel (Switzerland): S Karger; 1987. p. 169–71.

[5] Harsh G, Edwards M, Wilson C. Intracranial arachnoid cysts in children. J Neurosurg 1986; 64:835–42.

[6] French B. The embryology of spinal dysraphism. Clin Neurosurg 1983;30:295–340.

[7] Pang D. Split cord malformation: part II: clinical syndrome. J Neurosurg 1992;31:481–500.

[8] Barkovich A, Edwards M, Cogen P. MR evaluation of spinal dermal sinus tracts in children. AJNR Am J Neuroradiol 1991;12:123–9.

[9] Okumura Y, Sakaki T, Hirabayashi H. Middle cranial fossa arachnoid cyst developing in infancy. Case report. J Neurosurg 1995;82:1075–7.

[10] Zhou Y, Xu X, Chen L, et al. A Pro25arg substitution in mouse Fgfr1 causes expression of Cbf1 and premature fusion of calvarium and sutures. Hum Mol Genet 2006;9: 2001–8.

[11] Delashaw J, Persing J, Jane J. Cranial deformation in craniosynostosis. A new explanation. Neurosurg Clin N Am 1991;2:611–20.

[12] Pattisapu J, Walker M, Myers C, et al. Use of helmets in positional molding. In: Marlin A, editor. Concepts in pediatric neurosurgery. Basel (Switzerland): S Karger; 1989. p. 178–84.

[13] Agrawal D, Steinbok P, Cochrane D. Diagnosis of isolated sagittal synostosis: are radiographic studies necessary. Childs Nerv Syst 2006;22:375–8.

[14] Boop F, Chadduck W, Shewmare K, et al. Outcome analysis of 85 patients undergoing the pi procedure for correction of sagittal synostosis. J Neurosurg 1996;85:50–5.

[15] Kanev P, Lo A. Surgical correction of sagittal craniosynostosis: the morbidity of the pi procedure. J Craniofacial Surg 1995;6:98–102.

[16] Tessier P, Guiot G, Rougerie J, et al. Hypertelorism: cranionaso-orbito-facial and subethmoid osteotomy. Ann Chir Plast 1967;12:103–18.

[17] Goldstein J, Quereshy F, Cohen A. Early experience with biodegradeable fixation for congenital pediatric craniofacial surgery. J Craniofac Surg 1997;8:110–5.

[18] Jiminez D, Barone C. Endoscopy craniectomy for early surgical correction of sagittal craniosynostosis. J Neurosurg 1998;88:77–81.

[19] Fearon J, McLaughlin E, Kolar J. Sagittal craniosynostosis: surgical outcomes and long term growth. Plast Reconstr Surg 2006;117:532–41.

[20] Gindi S, Fairburn B. Intramedullary spinal abscess as a complication of a congenital dermal sinus. J Neurosurg 1969;30:484–97.

[21] Berger M, Wilson C. Posterior fossa epidermoid cysts. J Neurosurg 1985;62:214–9.

[22] Simpson D, David D, White J. Cephaoloceles: treatment, outcome and antenatal diagnosis. J Neurosurg 1984;15:14–21.

[23] Castillo M, Quencher R, Dominguez R. Chiari III malformation: imaging features. AJNR Am J Neuroradiol 1992;13:107–13.

[24] Crandall B, Chua C. Detecting neural tube defects by amniocentesis between 11 and 15 weeks gestation. Prenat Diagn 1985;15:339–43.

[25] McComb J. Spinal and cranial neural tube defects. Semin Pediatr Neurol 1997;4:156–66.

[26] Di Rocco C, Caldarelli M, Ceddia A. Incidence, anatomical distribution, and classification of arachnoidal cysts. In: Raimondi A, Choux M, Di Rocco C, editors. Intracranial cyst lesions. New York: Springer-Verlag; 1993. p. 101–11.

[27] Parsch C, Kraub J, Hoffman E, et al. Arachnoid cysts associated with subdural hematomas. Analysis of 16 cases, long-term follow-up and review of the literature. J Neurosurg 1997;40: 483–90.

[28] Yamanouchi Y, Someda K, Oka N. Spontaneous disappearance of middle fossa arachnoid cyst after head injury. Childs Nerv Syst 1986;2:40–3.

[29] Santamarta D, Arguas J, Ferrer E. The natural history of arachnoid cysts: endoscopic and cine-mode MRI evidence of a slit-valve mechanism. Minim Invasive Neurosurg 1995;38: 133–7.

[30] Rengachary S, Watanabe T. Ultrastructure and pathogenesis of intracranial arachnoid cysts. J Neuropathol Exp Neurol 1981;40:616–63.

[31] Shroeder H, Gaab M, Niendorf W. Neuroendoscopic approach to arachnoid cysts. J Neurosurg 1996;85:293–8.

[32] Galassi E, Piazza G. Arachnoid cysts of the middle cranial fossa: a clinical and radiological study of 25 cases treated surgically. Surg Neurol 1980;14:211–9.

[33] Galassi E, Gaist G, Giulani G, et al. Arachnoid cysts of the middle cranial fossa: experience with 77 cases treated surgically. Acta Neurochir 1988;42:201–7.

ELSEVIER
SAUNDERS

Otolaryngol Clin N Am
40 (2007) 27–60

OTOLARYNGOLOGIC
CLINICS
OF NORTH AMERICA

Cleft Lip and Palate

Oneida A. Arosarena, MD

Department of Otolaryngology, Temple University School of Medicine,
3400 North Broad Street, Kresge First Floor, Suite 102, Philadelphia, PA 19140, USA

Orofacial clefts are the most common craniofacial birth defects, second only to clubfoot in frequency of major birth anomalies [1]. Patients who have cleft lip or palate face significant lifelong communicative and aesthetic challenges, and difficulties with deglutition. The complex medical, ancillary, and psychosocial interactions necessary in the management of these patients warrants a multidisciplinary team approach [2]. Care of the cleft patient can be both challenging and rewarding.

Epidemiology

The overall incidence of orofacial clefting is typically quoted as 1 in 700 live births [3–5]. Cleft lip, with or without cleft palate (CL[P]), is an epidemiologically and etiologically distinct entity from isolated cleft palate (CP) [3,6]. Cleft lip is associated with cleft palate in 68% to 86% of cases [7]. The incidence of CL(P) varies significantly by racial group and with socioeconomic status, with an incidence of 1 in 1,000 births in whites, 1 in 500 births in Asians and Native Americans, and approximately 1 in 2,400 to 2,500 births in people of African descent [3,7]. The incidence of CP does not have the same ethnic heterogeneity and is typically quoted as 1 in 1,500 to 2,000 live births [4,5,7]. Between 60% and 80% of CL(P) patients are male, but a predominance of female infants affected by isolated cleft palate has been recognized [1,4,5,7]. Unilateral CL(P) is twice as common as bilateral CL(P), and usually affects the left side [7].

Causative factors

Although most children who have orofacial clefts are otherwise normal, the proportion of affected individuals who have recognized patterns of

E-mail address: oneida.arosarena@temple.edu

oto.theclinics.com

malformation has increased steadily over the years as cleft teams have incorporated the services of geneticists and dysmorphologists (Tables 1 and 2). More than 300 syndromes are known to be associated with orofacial clefting, but CP is more likely to be syndromic than CL(P). Approximately 14% to 30% of CL(P) cases are associated with multiple anomalies compared with 42% to 54% of CP cases [3,6–8].

The cause of isolated orofacial clefting is believed to be multifactorial [1]. Although clefting tends to cluster in families, its inheritance is not usually Mendelian and the discordance rate in monozygotic twins can be between 40% and 60% [4,6]. Several growth and transcription factors, receptors, polarizing signals, vasoactive peptides, cell adhesion proteins, extracellular matrix components, and matrix metalloproteinases are involved in palatal development. These biomolecules are expressed in a tightly controlled complex cascade, disturbance of which can result in orofacial clefting [5]. CL(P) has been associated with defects in the genetic loci for growth and transcription factors transforming growth factor-alpha (TGF-α), TGF-β2, TGF-β3, interferon regulatory factor-6 (van der Woude and popliteal pterygia syndromes), T-BOX 22 (X-linked cleft palate with ankyloglossia), P63

Table 1

Multiple malformation syndromes associated with cleft lip with or without cleft palate

Genetic disorders	Recognized patterns with unknown genesis	Teratogens[a]
Down syndrome	Amniotic band sequence	Anticonvulsant phenotype
Smith-Lemli-Opitz syndrome	Aicardi syndrome	Fetal alcohol syndrome
Aarskog syndrome	Kabuki make-up syndrome	Maternal diabetes
Coffin-Siris syndrome	Craniofrontonasal dysplasia	Maternal smoking
van der Woude syndrome	Hypertelorism microtia clefting syndrome	Maternal folate deficiency
Waardenburg syndrome	Focal dermal hypoplasia syndrome	—
Ectodermal dysplasia syndromes (Ectrodactyly-ectodermal dysplasia-clefting, Hay-Wells, and Rapp-Hodgkin syndromes)	—	—
Distal arthrogryposis type 2	—	—
Fryns syndrome	—	—
Popliteal pterygium syndrome	—	—
22q deletion syndromes (DiGeorge syndrome, Shprintzen syndrome, and CHARGE association)	—	—
Wolf-Hirschhorn syndrome	—	—
Basal cell nevus syndrome	—	—
Kallman syndrome	—	—
Nail patella syndrome	—	—

[a] Indicates increased risk rather than direct causation [3,6,11–13].

Table 2
Multiple malformation syndromes associated with cleft palate

Genetic disorders	Recognized patterns with unknown genesis	Teratogens[a]
Down syndrome	Pierre-Robin sequence	Anticonvulsant phenotype
Prader-Willi syndrome	Goldenhar syndrome	Fetal alcohol syndrome
Camptomelic dysplasia	Kabuki make-up syndrome	Thalidomide
Stickler syndrome	Mobius sequence	Dioxin
Holoprosencephaly	Klippel-Feil syndrome	Maternal smoking
de Lange syndrome	Silver-Russell syndrome	—
Spondyloepiphyseal dysplasia congenita	Beckwith-Wiedemann syndrome	—
Treacher-Collins syndrome	—	—
Cleft palate–short stature syndrome	—	—
22q deletion syndromes (DiGeorge syndrome, Shprintzen syndrome, and CHARGE association)	—	—
Diastrophic dysplasia	—	—
Orofaciodigital syndrome type I	—	—
Otopalatodigital syndrome type I	—	—
Limb mammary syndrome	—	—
Nager syndrome	—	—
Smith-Lemli-Opitz syndrome	—	—
X-linked cleft palate with ankyloglossia	—	—
Apert syndrome	—	—
Marfan syndrome	—	—
Turner syndrome	—	—
Cleidocranial dysostosis	—	—

[a] Indicates increased risk rather than direct causation [3,6,9,10,56–58].

(ectodermal dysplasia syndromes), Msx1, and the goosecoid transcription factor; for the vasoactive peptide endothelin-1 (22q deletion syndromes); for the retinoic acid receptor-alpha and the fibroblast growth factor receptor-1 (Kallman syndrome); for the cell adhesion molecule nectin-1 (ectodermal dysplasia syndromes); and several other genes whose functions have not yet been elucidated [3,9–13]. Similarly, CP has been associated with defects in the genetic loci for TGF-α, TGF-β3, T-BOX 22, and P63 (limb mammary syndrome); for the polarizing factor sonic hedgehog (holoprosencephaly); and the extracellular matrix proteins collagen type II and procollagen type XI (Stickler syndrome) [5,9,10,14]. Single gene disorders are believed to cause only 15% of clefts. The phenotypic heterogeneity demonstrated in the single gene disorders and variable penetrance, even in monozygotic twins, suggest that environmental factors also contribute to orofacial clefting. The role of epigenetic influences, such as maternal smoking, maternal alcohol use, folate deficiency or disordered metabolism, steroid and statin use, and retinoid exposure, is currently being investigated (see Tables 1 and 2) [9,10,13,15].

Embryology

Human facial development begins during the fourth week of intrauterine life when neural crest cells migrate and combine with the mesoderm to form the facial primordia [5]. The philtrum and primary palate (that portion of the palate and alveolus anterior to the incisive foramen) begin to form at approximately 35 days' gestational age by the coalition, growth, and differentiation of three embryonic prominences or processes (Fig. 1). The central segment of the face, comprising the forehead, supraorbital ridges, nose, philtrum, and primary palate, is derived from the frontonasal process. The intermaxillary segment of the frontonasal process is itself formed by the fusion of the two medial nasal prominences. This intermaxillary segment gives rise to the philtrum and that portion of the maxilla that bears the incisor teeth [14]. During the fifth and sixth weeks of intrauterine development, medial growth of the maxillary prominences, derived from the first branchial arches, results in fusion of the medial nasal and maxillary prominences to form the upper lip and anterior alveolus. Failure of fusion results in cleft lip and alveolus.

Formation of the secondary palate follows that of the primary palate. The secondary palate (that portion of the palate posterior to the incisive foramen) forms through the fusion of two paired outgrowths of the maxillary prominences, the palatal shelves (Fig. 2). The palatal shelves appear during the sixth week of development as vertical projections into the oral cavity on either side of the tongue. During the seventh week, the shelves elevate, assume a horizontal orientation, and fuse, closing the secondary palate. This fusion begins at the incisive foramen, progresses toward the posterior palate, and is complete at about the 12th week of intrauterine life. Failure of fusion results in a cleft palate (Fig. 3). The severity of the palatal cleft varies from submucous clefting to complete bilateral clefting extending to the maxillary alveolus [16]. Although the tongue does not participate in palatal closure in the normal situation, altered tongue position may mechanically block fusion of the palatal shelves, as in the Robin sequence. The tongue musculature is known to become functional at about the time of palatal shelf elevation [14].

Preoperative assessment

Initial assessment and identification of associated anomalies

The initial assessment of the infant born with an orofacial cleft includes a birth history, thorough head and neck examination, and examination of the infant's extremities to identify associated malformations (see Tables 1

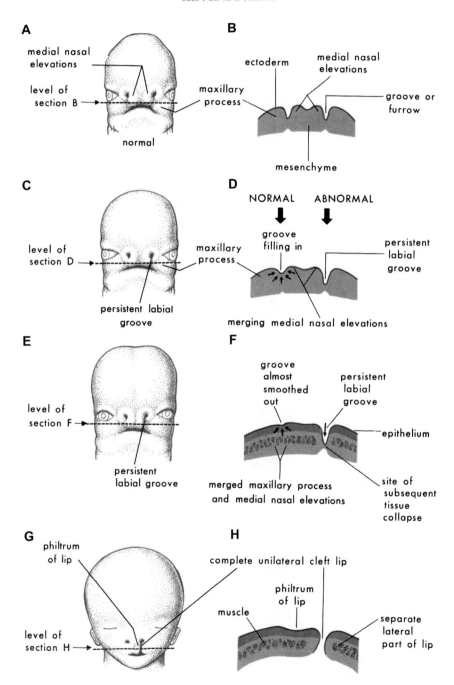

Fig. 1. (*A-H*) Intrauterine midfacial development, 5 weeks to 10 weeks. (*From* Moore KL. The branchial apparatus and the head and neck. In: Moore KL, editor. Before we are born: basic embryology and birth defects. 3rd edition. Philadelphia: WB Saunders; 1989. p. 134–58; with permission.)

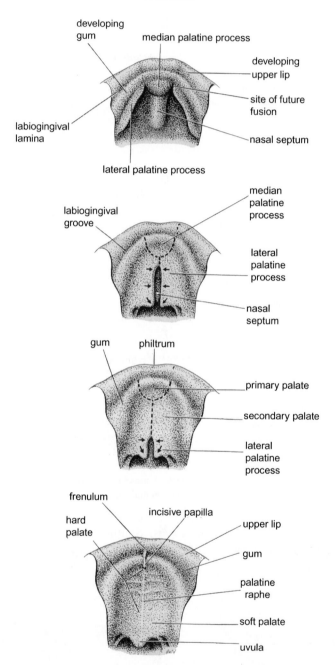

Fig. 2. Intrauterine development of secondary palate, 6 weeks to 12 weeks. (*From* Moore KL. The branchial apparatus and the head and neck. In: Moore KL, editor. Before we are born: basic embryology and birth defects. 3rd edition. Philadelphia: WB Saunders; 1989. p. 134–58; with permission.)

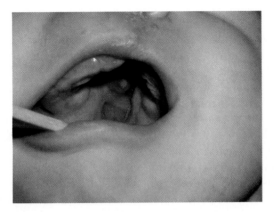

Fig. 3. Infant with complete unilateral cleft palate.

and 2). A history of intrauterine growth retardation may indicate Smith-Lemli-Opitz or Wolf-Hirschhorn syndrome. Down-slanting lateral canthi may indicate Treacher-Collins or Aarskog syndrome, whereas up-slanting lateral canthi and epicanthal folds indicate Down or Smith-Lemli-Opitz syndrome. Down-slanting lateral canthi with hypertelorism, blepharoptosis, epicanthal folds and colobomata are physical signs present in Wolf-Hirschhorn syndrome. Hypertelorism, blepharoptosis, and a simian crease are also characteristic of Aarskog syndrome. Ankyloblepharon with entropion and absent eyelashes indicate Hay-Wells syndrome.

Auricular abnormalities can occur with any of the 22q deletion syndromes and Treacher-Collins syndrome. Unilateral microtia or anotia with hemifacial microsomia typifies Goldenhar syndrome. An enlarged, cauliflower, or calcified auricle, and associated laryngotracheomalacia suggest diastrophic dysplasia.

CL(P) or CP with lower lip pits is pathognomonic for van der Woude syndrome. A grimace should be elicited to assess facial nerve function to rule out Mobius sequence. Digital malformations or agenesis characterize Aarskog, Coffin-Siris, de Lange, Nager, Fryns, Smith-Lemli-Opitz, Silver-Russell, limb mammary, ectrodactyly-ectodermal dysplasia-clefting and otopalatodigital syndromes, and amnion rupture sequence [1,6,11]. Patients who have orofaciodigital syndrome manifest hamartomas or lipomas of the tongue and digital malformations. Infants who have Robin sequence, otopalatodigital syndrome, Nager syndrome, Smith-Lemli-Opitz syndrome, Kabuki syndrome, Silver-Russell syndrome, and Stickler syndrome have characteristic micrognathia [9,17,18]. As upper airway compromise complicates several of the syndromes associated with CP, these patients may require immediate stabilization by positioning, tongue-lip adhesion, mandibular distraction, or tracheotomy in severe cases before palatal repair. Certainly, children who have cleft with other malformations should be referred with their families to the cleft team geneticist or dysmorphologist [19].

Feeding

The most immediate concern in the care of the infant who has cleft, other than the airway, is nutrition. The extent of the cleft often correlates with the infant's ability to feed. Patients who have clefts limited to the soft palate usually have normal sucking, whereas infants who have hard palate clefts are often unable to generate the negative pressure needed for normal sucking because of the oronasal communication. Impaired sucking can lead to weight loss and failure to thrive as the infant expends more energy in feeding than he or she is able to ingest.

Early swallowing therapy is required in the infant who has a complete CP to ensure near-normal feeding and growth. Parents can be taught to use squeeze bottles with cross-cut nipples to increase the flow of formula in concert with the infant's suck. In general, most newborns who have clefts should be able to ingest 2 to 3 ounces of formula with assistance within 20 to 30 minutes. Frequent burping is required during feeding because of aerophagia. Alternatively, bottles with nipples specialized for CP feeding, such as the Haberman feeder, can be used to limit air ingestion. Frequent assessments by the cleft team speech and swallowing pathologist may be needed to establish parental confidence in feeding. Patients who fail to gain weight or demonstrate excessive aerophagia may require placement of a palatal obturator by the cleft team pedodontist. Patients who have CL(P) and associated protruding premaxillae, particularly those who have bilateral clefts, should undergo lip adhesion or premaxillary orthopedics at approximately age 12 weeks. Lip adhesion not only decreases the size of the palatal cleft by normalizing the position of the premaxilla, but also restores the sphincter function of the orbicularis oris, which improves feeding. Monthly assessments by the facial plastic surgeon are recommended to evaluate patient growth and development, and more frequent follow-up by the cleft team pediatrician may be needed in patients who have failure to thrive or developmental delay.

Otolaryngologic assessment

The abnormal insertion of the tensor veli palatini is believed to contribute to Eustachian tube dysfunction, middle ear disease, and the conductive hearing loss associated with CP. The placement of myringotomy tubes is routine at the time of CP repair [7,20]. Because several multiple malformation syndromes associated with clefting (eg, Stickler syndrome, van der Woude syndrome, Klippel-Fiel syndrome, Waardenburg syndrome, Down syndrome, and diastrophic dysplasia) also manifest sensorineural hearing loss, hearing assessment by auditory brainstem response testing or other methods should be performed in the first months of life.

Psychosocial support

Families of infants who have clefts require counseling by a cleft team social worker or psychologist as they adjust to the stresses of caring for the infant and frequent interaction with medical professionals. This is particularly true of families whose infants were not diagnosed with a cleft while in utero, who have limited resources or support, or who have infants who have multiple anomalies. Stages of shock, denial, sadness, anger, and adaptation and reorganization have been described in parents of infants who have clefts [21].

Unilateral cleft lip

Anatomy

The cleft lip deformity results from deficiency and displacement of soft tissues, cartilage, and bone in the area of the cleft [7]. The principle muscle of the lip is the orbicularis oris, which interdigitates with the other mimetic muscles of the midface and lower face (Fig. 4A) [20]. In the cleft lip, there is discontinuity of the orbicularis oris in the region of the cleft, and the fibers of the orbicularis parallel the cleft margin, inserting on the alar base on the

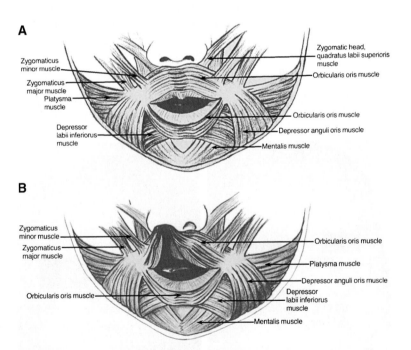

Fig. 4. (*A*) Mimetic muscles of the lower face. (*From* Sykes J, Senders C. Pathologic anatomy of cleft lip, palate, and nasal deformities. In: Meyers AD, editor. Biological basis of facial plastic surgery. New York: Thieme Medical Publishers; 1993. p. 59; with permission.) (*B*) Abnormal insertion of orbicularis oris in cleft lip. (*From* Sykes J, Senders C. Pathologic anatomy of cleft lip, palate, and nasal deformities. In: Meyers AD, editor. Biological basis of facial plastic surgery. New York: Thieme Medical Publishers; 1993. p. 61; with permission.)

lateral side of the cleft, and on the columellar base and septum on the medial side of the cleft (Fig. 4B) [7,19,20]. Moreover, the orbicularis oris is hypoplastic in the area of the cleft [20,22].

The abnormal muscular forces and maxillary osseous discontinuity result in an outward rotation of the premaxillary-bearing medial segment and retrodisplacement of the lateral segment (Fig. 5A). The muscular attachment to the caudal septum is also believed to result in its displacement out of the vomerine groove and into the noncleft nostril, which in turn results in shortening of the columella. The philtrum is short on the cleft side, the peak of Cupid's bow is rotated superiorly, and the vermilion is also deficient in the region of the cleft. In the nasal tip, the domes are separated and the lateral crus is flattened on the cleft side [7].

The severity of cleft lip varies from clefts involving only the vermilion to full-thickness clefts involving all tissue layers. A malformation consisting of dehiscence of the orbicularis muscle with vermilion notching but intact overlying skin is termed a microform cleft [7,20]. An incomplete cleft lip spares some of the superior portion of the upper lip. Anatomic dissections on stillborn infants reveal that the orbicularis oris muscle in the incomplete cleft lip does not cross the cleft unless the cutaneous bridge is at least one third of the height of the lip. Moreover, the orientation of the small amount of muscle that bridges the cleft in this situation is abnormal [20,23].

Timing of cleft lip repair

Generally, cleft lip repair with primary tip rhinoplasty is performed at age 3 months. The patient's overall health status, including the presence of other

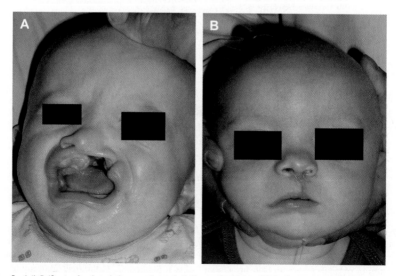

Fig. 5. (*A*) Infant who has left complete cleft lip and palate. (*B*) Infant 1 month after rotation-advancement repair and primary tip rhinoplasty. Note stenosis of nostril on left.

congenital anomalies, may dictate that repair of the cleft be delayed, however. Widely followed preoperative guidelines include the rules of ten: weight at least 10 pounds, hemoglobin at least 10 g, white blood cell count less than $10,000/mm^3$, and age more than 10 weeks [7,20,24]. Patients who have wide complete unilateral clefts or bilateral clefts with marked premaxillary protrusion may require staged repair with lip adhesion performed at age 3 months and definitive repair performed at age 5 to 6 months. When lip adhesion includes muscular repair across the cleft (eg, a Rose-Thompson straight-line repair), it has the advantage of increasing the length of the cutaneous portion of the lip, which facilitates the definitive repair. Alternatively, presurgical maxillary orthopedics may be used before lip repair in the case of the wide cleft, but is associated with increased cost and burden of treatment [7,25,26]. Lip adhesion may also be used with a passive molding device to prevent collapse of the alveolar arch form [27].

Cheiloplasty techniques for the unilateral cleft lip

The first documentation of cleft lip repair occurred in the fourth century AD in China. This simple technique involved freshening and approximation of the cut cleft edges, and remained the standard of care until 1825 when von Graefe proposed the use of curved incisions to allow lengthening of the lip. His work provided the foundation for the Rose-Thompson technique and other straight-line closure repairs introduced in the early 1900s [7,20]. The straight-line closures, however, had the disadvantage of vertical scar contracture leading to notching of the lip [20].

Several methods were developed to avert the scar contracture associated with the straight-line closures. These included numerous geometric repairs that were also designed to irregularize the lip scar [20]. In the 1950s, Tennison and Randall introduced a triangular flap that created a Z-plasty in the lower portion of the lip scar. All of these techniques produced scars that violated the philtrum, however [7,20].

The Millard rotation-advancement technique, introduced in 1957, is the most widely used procedure for cleft lip repair because it places most of the scar along the natural philtral border and is more flexible than the geometric closures. Moreover, the Millard technique allows for complete muscular repair and primary cleft rhinoplasty, and minimizes the discarding of normal tissue. Its disadvantages include the need for extensive undermining and the risk for nostril stenosis on the cleft side (Fig. 5B) [20]. The author's modification of the technique is described below.

Surgical technique
Flap design. Commonly used reference points for flap design are illustrated in Fig. 6 and described as follows [20]:

Point 1: Center or low point of Cupid's bow
Point 2: Peak of Cupid's bow on noncleft side

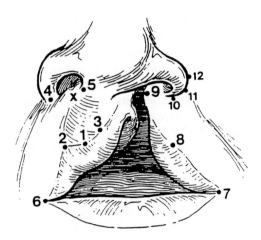

Fig. 6. Reference points for Millard rotation-advancement technique for unilateral cleft lip repair. (*From* Ness JA, Sykes JM. Basics of Millard rotation-advancement technique for repair of the unilateral cleft lip deformity. Facial Plast Surg 1993;9:169; with permission.)

Point 3: Peak of Cupid's bow, medial side of cleft
Point 4: Alar base, noncleft side
Point 5: Columellar base, noncleft side
Point 6: Commissure, noncleft side
Point 7: Commissure, cleft side
Point 8: Peak of Cupid's bow, lateral side of cleft
Point 9: Superior extent of advancement flap
Point 10: Alar base, cleft side
Point x: Back-cut point

The following measurements are made to ensure accuracy in marking the reference points [20]:

1 to 2 = 1 to 3 = 2–4 mm
2 to 6 = 8 to 7 ≈ 20 mm
2 to 4 = 8 to 10 = 9–11 mm
3 to 5 + x = 8 to 9

Flap elevation. After the induction of general anesthesia, the patient is intubated with an oral RAE tube. The reference points are marked, and the patient's lip is infiltrated with a few milliliters of local anesthetic with 1:200,000 epinephrine as a field block at the oral commissures to prevent distortion of the lip anatomy near the cleft. The rotation incision is marked from point x to point 5 to point 3. A full-thickness rotation incision is made and extended into the red lip to the wet line.

The advancement flap is elevated by incising along the vermilion-cutaneous junction from the height of Cupid's bow medially (from point 8 to point 9, see Fig. 6) on the lateral margin of the cleft. This incision is also extended into the red lip to the wet line (Fig. 7). The skin is elevated off of the orbicularis oris muscle for approximately 1 cm on both sides of the cleft. Bilateral gingivolabial sulcus incisions are made, which extend to the cleft margins. The soft tissues of the lip and cheek are elevated off of the maxilla in a supraperiosteal plane, using blunt dissection and preserving the infraorbital nerves. This elevation may continue as superiorly as the level of the nasal bones to allow maximal flap advancement and rotation, and tensionless closure if the cleft is wide. The orbicularis is freed from its abnormal attachments to the columellar base and alar margin on the lateral side of the cleft. The alar margin on the cleft side is released from its attachment to the piriform aperture using an internal alotomy [20]. The advancement flap elevation is completed by incising along the nasal sill (point 9 to point 10, see Fig. 6) but this incision may be extended to the alar facial groove if necessary (point 9 to point 11 or 12, see Fig. 6). The c-flap is elevated after incising along the vermilion-cutaneous junction from the height of Cupid's bow medially on the medial margin of the cleft (Fig. 7).

Closure. The intraoral mucosa is closed with dissolvable suture. The gingivolabial sulcus mucosa may be attached to the nasal spine to elevate the gingivolabial sulcus. The orbicularis oris is reconstituted across the cleft with semipermanent suture (Fig. 8). The alar base on the cleft side is medialized by placement of a subcutaneous stitch from the alar base to the periosteum of the nasal spine. The c-flap may be rotated into the nasal floor to prevent stenosis of the nostril on the cleft side, or it may be discarded. The skin closure in the nasal floor is performed with 6-0 monofilament fast-absorbing suture. The lip skin closure is performed with 5-0 monofilament subcuticular sutures (Fig. 9). The skin closure is reinforced with surgical skin tape.

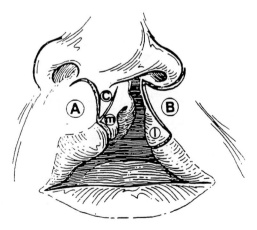

Fig. 7. Flaps in Millard rotation-advancement technique for unilateral cleft lip repair. (*From* Ness JA, Sykes JM. Basics of Millard rotation-advancement technique for repair of the unilateral cleft lip deformity. Facial Plast Surg 1993;9:171; with permission.)

AROSARENA

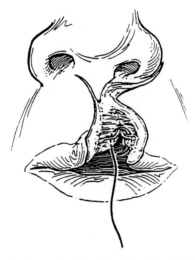

Fig. 8. Repair of orbicularis oris muscle. (*From* Ness JA, Sykes JM. Basics of Millard rotation-advancement technique for repair of the unilateral cleft lip deformity. Facial Plast Surg 1993;9:174; with permission.)

Tip rhinoplasty. Primary cleft rhinoplasty lessens the cleft nasal deformity [7,20,28]. Wide undermining of the nasal skin from the underlying nasal cartilages is performed either through the lip incision or an alar margin incision. The vestibular skin is not dissected from the alar cartilages to minimize the risk for alar stenosis [20]. The dome on the noncleft side is

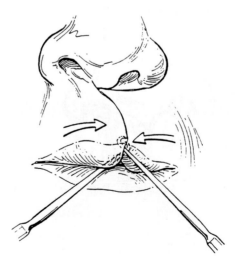

Fig. 9. Placement of rotation and advancement flaps. (*From* Ness JA, Sykes JM. Basics of Millard rotation-advancement technique for repair of the unilateral cleft lip deformity. Facial Plast Surg 1993;9:173; with permission.)

delivered, and the dome is recreated and elevated in the cleft alar cartilage using an interdomal suture. Alternatively, the dome on the cleft side may be repositioned with external bolsters [7,20]. If an alar margin incision is used, it is closed with 5-0 chromic gut suture. Arm splints are placed before the patient is awakened.

Bilateral cleft lip

Anatomy

In the bilateral cleft lip, the orbicularis oris muscle inserts on both alar margins, and no muscle fibers invade the prolabium. Unrestrained growth of the vomer and nasal septum result in protrusion of the premaxilla (Fig. 10) [7,26]. The prolabial skin is flat, lacking philtral ridges, a philtral dimple, and Cupid's bow. The columella is very short, and both lateral crura are flattened, resulting in alar flaring [7]. The advantage of the bilateral cleft lip is symmetry [29].

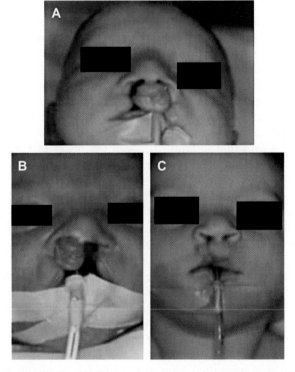

Fig. 10. (*A, B*) Infants who have bilateral cleft lip and maxillary protrusion; (*C*) Child in (*B*) following lip adhesion.

Cheiloplasty techniques for the bilateral cleft lip

Early bilateral cleft lip repair techniques involved excision of the premaxilla and prolabium, resulting in an unnatural appearance to the upper lip and deleterious effects on midfacial growth [7,26]. Later, premaxillary setback with vomerine osteotomies was popularized in the 1800s to manage premaxillary protrusion. This technique was also associated with significant midfacial growth hindrance, however [7,19]. Current bilateral cleft cheiloplasty techniques are modifications of Millard's bilateral straight-line repair. Modern principles that guide the repair of the bilateral cleft lip are [7,29]:

Symmetry
Primary muscular continuity
Proper philtral size and shape
Formation of the median tubercle from lateral lip elements
Primary positioning of alar cartilages to construct the nasal tip and
    columella

Surgical technique
Flap elevation. The patient's lip is infiltrated with local anesthetic with 1:200,000 epinephrine as a field block at the oral commissures to prevent distortion of the lip anatomy near the clefts. The prolabial skin is also infiltrated with a small amount of local anesthetic. The prolabial vermilion-cutaneous junction is incised. The mucosa of the prolabium is dissected from the premaxilla in a supraperiosteal plane, and is turned down to line the premaxillary gingivolabial sulcus.

The philtral flap is designed based on the child's ethnicity, with suggested dimensions of 6 to 8 mm of length, 2 mm of width at the columellar-labial junction, and 3 to 4 mm of width between the peaks of Cupid's bow for Caucasians. These measurements are based on Mulliken and colleagues' [30] prospective anthropometric study of 46 Caucasian children who had bilateral clefts who were compared with normal children. Slightly wider philtral flaps are used for children of other ethnicities, but these flaps should rarely exceed 5 to 6 mm in width [7,30]. Because of the tendency for the philtrum to widen in children who have bilateral clefts, Mulliken's philtral flaps are designed with concave sides and a dart-shaped tip (Fig. 11) [29]. The remainder of the prolabial skin may be discarded, or flanking strips of skin may be deepithelialized on each side of the philtral flap for additional height to re-create the philtral ridges [25,29]. In addition, small bilateral c-flaps may be designed to line the nasal floor. The prolabial skin is elevated in a supraperiosteal plane to the level of the nasal spine.

The advancement flaps are elevated by incising along the vermilion-cutaneous junction from the height of Cupid's bow medially on the lateral lip elements. These incisions are extended into the red lip to the wet line.

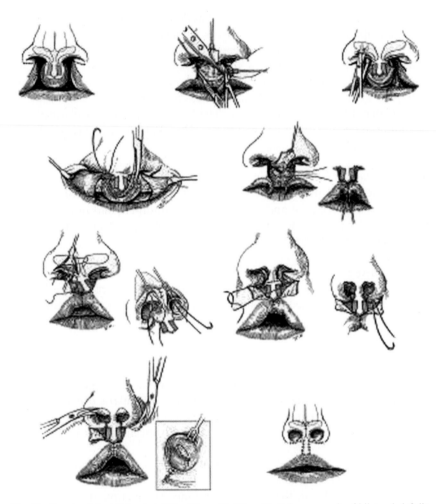

Fig. 11. Repair of the bilateral cleft lip. (*From* Mulliken JB. Primary repair of bilateral cleft lip and nasal deformity. Plast Reconstr Surg 2001;108:186; with permission.)

The mucosal flaps created by these incisions along the cleft margins are dissected supraperiosteally, and sutured to the prolabial mucosa with absorbable suture, thus effecting bilateral gingivoperiosteoplasty.

The skin is elevated off of the orbicularis oris muscle for approximately 1 cm on the lateral elements of the cleft. Bilateral gingivolabial sulcus incisions are made, which extend to the cleft margins. As with repair of the unilateral cleft lip, the soft tissues of the lip and cheek are elevated off the maxilla in a supraperiosteal plane. The orbicularis is freed from its abnormal attachments to the alar margins using internal alotomies [20]. Elevation of the advancement flaps is completed by incising along the nasal sills.

Closure. The intraoral mucosa is closed as described for repair of the unilateral cleft lip, and the orbicularis oris is reconstituted across the cleft. The alar bases are medialized by placement of subcutaneous stitches from the alar bases to the periosteum of the nasal spine. The dermis of each alar base is sutured to the underlying muscle to prevent alar elevation with smiling [29]. The skin closure in the bilateral nasal floor is performed with 6-0 monofilament fast-absorbing suture. The lip skin closure is performed with 5-0 monofilament subcuticular sutures. The skin closures are reinforced with surgical skin tape.

Tip rhinoplasty. The nasal correction is performed through alar rim incisions as described previously for the unilateral cleft nasal deformity. The alar domes are recreated and elevated using intradomal and interdomal sutures. The alar margin incisions are closed and arm splints are placed before the patient is awakened.

Postoperative care

After cleft lip repair, the patient is hospitalized until oral intake is sufficient. Feeding is resumed with a syringe or cup. Arm splints are maintained for the first two postoperative weeks to prevent patient disruption of the lip repair.

Complications and their management

Notch in the vermilion. This complication indicates incomplete muscular repair or dehiscence of the inferior portion of the orbicularis oris repair. It is corrected by reapproximation of the lowest portion of the lip muscle. The overlying mucosa may be excised, or a V-Y advancement performed.

Malalignment of Cupid's bow or whistle deformity. This condition is frequently caused by contracture of the lip scar, and can be prevented by placement of a Z-plasty at the vermilion-cutaneous junction during primary cheiloplasty. The scar may be excised secondarily, and the vermilion correctly repositioned with a Z-plasty to prevent recurrence of the deformity.

Absence of the median tubercle and part of Cupid's bow. Commonly seen after bilateral cleft lip repair, this problem is difficult to correct. Paired vermilion-orbicularis flaps may be used to correct this deformity, or a cross lip flap may be necessary [7,31].

Cleft palate

Anatomy

The normal palate consists of a bony anterior component and a posterior soft-tissue component. Normal mobility of the soft palate is essential for speech and swallowing function. This mobility depends on six paired muscles that normally insert on the soft palate (Fig. 12A):

Levator veli palatini
Musculus uvulus
Superior constrictor
Palatopharyngeus
Palatoglossus
Tensor veli palatini

Of the six, the muscles that seem to have the greatest impact on velopharyngeal competence are the levator, the uvulus, and the superior constrictor. The levator veli palatini pulls the soft palate, or velum, superiorly and posteriorly, allowing it to appose the posterior pharyngeal wall. The musculus

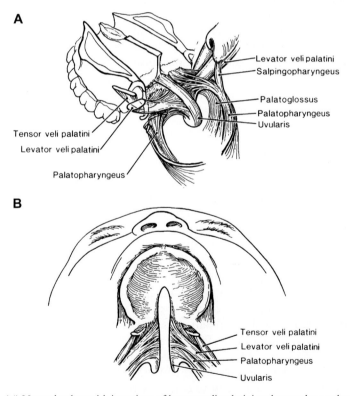

Fig. 12. (*A*) Normal palate with insertions of levator veli palatini and musculus uvulus on midline tensor aponeurosis. (*From* Senders CW, Sykes JM. Cleft palate. In: Smith JD, Bumsted RM, editors. Pediatric facial plastic and reconstructive surgery. New York: Raven Press; 1993. p. 162; with permission.) (*B*) Cleft palate demonstrating insertion of levator on posterior edge of hard palate and on edges of cleft. (*From* Senders CW, Sykes JM. Cleft palate. In: Smith JD, Bumsted RM, editors. Pediatric facial plastic and reconstructive surgery. New York: Raven Press; 1993. p. 163; with permission.)

uvulus increases the bulk of the velum during its contraction, aiding in closure of the oropharyngeal-nasopharyngeal communication. The superior constrictor is responsible for the sphincter function of the pharynx, moving the pharyngeal walls medially during phonation and swallowing [4]. This sphincter function can become critical in patients who have marginal velar length or function who may compensate for their velar insufficiency with hypermobility of the superior constrictor. The palatopharyngeus may also play a role in medialization of the pharyngeal wall and causes downward displacement of the palate. The palatoglossus is also a palatal depressor that is believed to be responsible for the production of nasal phonemes by allowing controlled passage of air to the nasal chamber [4]. Both the palatopharyngeus and palatoglossus play important roles in swallowing. The tensor moderates patency of the Eustachian tube.

In the cleft palate, the aponeurosis of the tensor veli palatini inserts onto the bony edges of the cleft, rather than onto its normal insertion on the posterior edge of the hard palate (Fig. 12B). Both the levator and tensor normally insert on the palatal aponeurosis. In the cleft palate the levator sling is interrupted by insertion of the muscle onto the posterior edge of the hard palate [1,4]. The function of the tensor is also compromised because of its abnormal insertion, leading to inadequate ventilation of the middle ear space. Because the aponeurotic attachment is more anterior in the cleft palate, the cleft palate is shorter than the normal palate [1,4].

Pathophysiology

The speech pathology associated with unrepaired cleft palate consists of two components. The primary component of cleft speech pathology is directly related to the oronasal communication, and is corrected surgically. It consists of velopharyngeal dysfunction, hypernasality, and nasal air escape. Velopharyngeal dysfunction refers to the inability of the soft palate to appose the posterior pharyngeal wall and close the nasopharyngeal-oropharyngeal communication during speech and swallowing. The sufficiency of the velum depends on its length (adequacy) and muscular function (competence).

The secondary component of cleft speech pathology is a learned or compensatory response in the unrepaired cleft palate or in the repaired palate with an oronasal fistula or dysfunctional velum. This response consists of glottal stops, pharyngeal fricatives, consonant substitutions, and decreased consonant range that are carryovers from the child's structural constraints in early infancy and are difficult to correct with speech therapy. Such misarticulations are best prevented by completing palatal repair by age 12 months [1,4,32–34].

The goals of cleft palate therapy and repair are to:

Separate the oral and nasal cavities to prevent reflux of the food bolus into the nares and promote nasal hygiene.

Normalize swallowing physiology by obliterating the oronasal communication and reconstructing a palate with a functional velum that has adequate length.

Promote normal or near-normal speech by repair of the palatal cleft and
speech therapeutic intervention, while limiting the negative effects of
cleft palate repair on midfacial growth.

Perform mucoperiosteal repair of the cleft alveolus to correct anterior oronasal communication and facilitate possible bone growth across the
alveolar cleft, thus preventing tooth loss.

Timing of cleft palate repair

Despite the publication of numerous series on outcomes of cleft palate
repair, considerable controversy still exists as to the timing of cleft palate
and cleft alveolar repair. Many surgeons continue to advocate two-stage repair of the cleft palate to limit the effects of hard palatal repair on maxillary
growth. Mucoperiosteal repair of the hard palate cleft is known to result in
subperiosteal scarring. Because midfacial growth occurs by bone deposition
by the hard palate periosteal osteocytes with concomitant osteoclastic bone
resorption along the nasal floor and in the maxillary sinuses, subperiosteal
scarring impairs midfacial growth. This midfacial growth impedance results
in a prognathic profile (Fig. 13). Advocates of two-stage palatal repair perform repair of the soft palate between 3 and 8 months of age while delaying

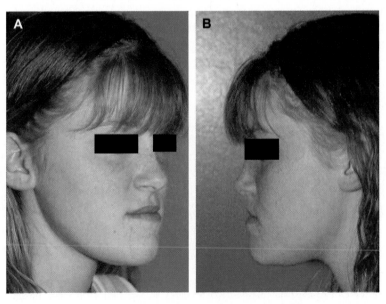

Fig. 13. (*A, B*) Teenaged patient with midfacial hypoplasia resulting from cleft palate repair in
infancy.

hard palate repair until 15 months to 15 years of age. No significant difference in craniofacial morphology has been identified in children who had palatal clefts repaired between age 8 months and 8 years [35–37]. If hard palate closure is delayed until full facial growth has been attained, however, this distortion is nearly eliminated at the expense of abnormal speech, which may be difficult to correct [4,26,37,38]. Nevertheless, most craniofacial surgeons advocate complete repair of palatal clefts between age 9 and 12 months to prevent the detrimental effects of delayed repair on speech and language development [2,4,7,34].

Palatoplasty techniques

The management of the CP has evolved from obturation in the 1700s; to simple repairs of the cleft soft palate in the early 1800s; to two-flap complete palatal repairs, such as von Langenbeck's palatoplasty in the late 1800s (Fig. 14); to repairs that lengthen the palate, such as the Veau-Wardill-Kilner V-to-Y advancement technique in the 1930s (Fig. 15); to repairs that not only close the palatal cleft and lengthen the palate but also correctly align the palatal musculature (Table 3) [4]. Recreation of the levator sling during CP repair has been associated with a higher probability of successful speech development [7,39]. In their comparison study of Furlow palatoplasty and von Langenbeck palatoplasty patients, Yu and colleagues [40] found 98% of the patients who had undergone Furlow palatoplasty had velopharyngeal adequacy and excellent speech compared with 70% of the von Langenbeck palatoplasty patients. The surgical technique selected for CP repair depends on the extent of the cleft, and whether or not the cleft is unilateral or bilateral.

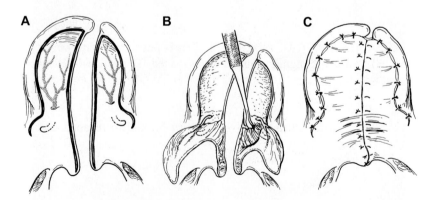

Fig. 14. (*A-C*) Two-flap palatoplasty. (*From* Senders CW, Sykes JM. Cleft palate. In: Smith JD, Bumsted RM, editors. Pediatric facial plastic and reconstructive surgery. New York: Raven Press; 1993. p. 167; with permission.)

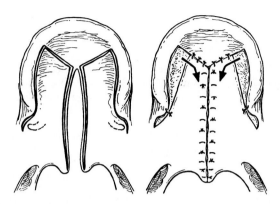

Fig. 15. Push-back palatoplasty. (*From* Senders CW, Sykes JM. Cleft palate. In: Smith JD, Bumsted RM, editors. Pediatric facial plastic and reconstructive surgery. New York: Raven Press; 1993. p. 165; with permission.)

Clefts limited to the soft palate

Although soft palate clefts can be simply closed by incising along the cleft edges and reapproximating the nasopharyngeal mucosa and oral mucosa in the midline, this technique does not easily allow for muscular repair, as the muscle attaches on the posterior margin of the hard palate. Moreover, this method does not increase palatal length, and the scar contracture of the straight-line closure may even shorten the velum. For these reasons, the author's preferred method of soft palate cleft repair is the Furlow double opposing Z-plasty, which concurrently lengthens the palate and correctly re-aligns the levator veli palatini. Long-term studies have demonstrated improved speech results and reduced rates of secondary surgery for correction of velopharyngeal dysfunction when comparing the double opposing Z-plasty to other palatoplasty methods [7,40].

Surgical technique. After the induction of general anesthesia, the patient is intubated with an oral RAE tube. The patient is positioned with his or her neck extended, and a Dingman tongue gag is placed. The soft palate mucosa is injected with 0.5% lidocaine with 1:200,000 epinephrine. It is important to allow at least 10 minutes for the maximal vasoconstrictive effect of the epinephrine to limit blood loss in the infant. During this time, tympanostomy tube placement and/or intraoperative auditory brainstem response testing may be performed.

The incisions for flap design described herein are for the right-handed surgeon. The flap design may be reversed for the left-handed surgeon. The mucosa is incised along the medial edge of the cleft bilaterally. On the right side an incision is made along the posterior edge of the hard palate through the mucosa and the attachments of the levator veli palatini to the hard palate (Fig. 16). An oral mucosal flap is developed on the right side, keeping the

Table 3
Palatoplasty options

Technique	Advantages	Disadvantages
von Langenbeck's two-flap palatoplasty	Allows facile closure of alveolar cleft	Does not increase velar length Does not reorient levator sling Longitudinal scar contracture results in short palate Denudes palatal bone
Veau-Wardill-Kilner V-to-Y pushback palatoplasty	Provides some increased palatal length	Difficult to repair alveolar cleft with this technique Does not reorient levator sling Longitudinal scar contracture can limit palatal lengthening Denudes palatal bone
Furlow palatoplasty	Significantly lengthens velum Recreates levator sling Does not denude palatal bone Allows closure of alveolar cleft	Increased operative time compared to other methods Technically challenging Creates dead space between oral and nasal mucosa that fills with hematoma Increased risk for palatal fistulae with wide clefts Oral displacement of palatal mucosa may negatively affect speech
Combined two-flap/ Furlow palatoplasty	Significantly lengthens velum Recreates levator sling Allows closure of alveolar cleft	Increased operative time compared to other methods Technically challenging Denudes palatal bone

levator attached to the oral mucosa and separating it from the underlying nasal mucosa. Care is taken not to incise the nasal mucosa at this time. The oral mucosa is then elevated off the posterior edge of the hard palate for a few millimeters with care being taken to preserve the greater palatine neurovascular bundle. The soft tissue attachments to the pterygoid hamulus are divided, and the tensor palatini is elevated out of the hamulus. Although many surgeons describe fracturing of the hamulus to decrease tension on the palatal closure, fracturing of the hamulus has been associated with damage to the ascending palatine artery, which supplies the velar musculature [4,41]. The dissection then proceeds more laterally over the tensor into the space of Ernst between the superior constrictor muscle and the pterygoids. This dissection results in increased medial rotation of the flap. Starting at the posteromedial edge of the cleft, the mucosa is elevated from the nasal surface of the hard palate to allow mobilization of the nasal mucoperiosteum. The nasal mucosal flap on the right side is created by incising the nasal mucosa from the uvula to the torus tubarius. The dissected area on the right side can be packed with neurosurgical cottonoids soaked in 1:200,000 topical epinephrine to limit blood loss during dissection of the flaps on the left side.

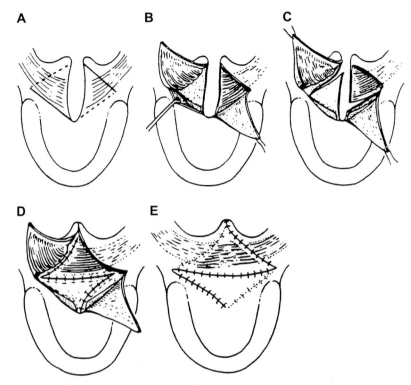

Fig. 16. (*A-E*) Double opposing Z-plasty soft palate cleft repair. (*From* Gage-White L. Furlow palatoplasty: double opposing Z-plasty. Facial Plast Surg 1993;9:181–3; with permission.)

On the left side, the oral mucosal flap is developed by incising the mucosa from the uvula to the maxillary tuberosity. The oral mucosa is then elevated off of the levator palatini, leaving the levator attached to the nasal mucosa. As with the right side, the oral mucosa is elevated off the posterior edge of the hard palate, the soft tissue attachments to the hamulus are divided, the tensor is elevated out of the hamulus, and the dissection is carried into the space of Ernst. The oral mucosal flap is retracted, and the nasal mucosal flap on the left side is created by detaching the nasal mucosa with the attached levator from the posterior edge of the hard palate. A small cuff of nasal mucosal tissue should be kept on the hard palate to facilitate closure.

At this point, closure of the palatoplasty begins by transposition of the nasal mucosal Z-plasty flaps. The nasal mucosal flap from the right side is sutured to the posterior hard palate nasal mucosa on the left side with absorbable suture. This closure begins adjacent to the left pterygoid hamulus and proceeds from left to right. The left nasal mucosal flap is then transposed and sutured to the mucosa at the base of the right pterygoid hamulus. This mucosal flap is then sutured to the previously transposed right nasal mucosal flap. A uvuloplasty is then performed before transposition of the oral mucosal flaps. The left oral mucosal flap is sutured to the mucosa of the right maxillary tuberosity and then to the mucosa of the posterior edge of the oral surface of the hard palate. The right oral mucosal flap is then transposed and sutured to the left maxillary tuberosity and the previously transposed left oral mucosal flap, completing the closure. The oral cavity, oropharynx, nares, and nasopharynx are copiously irrigated and suctioned. Arm splints are placed before the patient is awakened.

Unilateral complete cleft palate

Although some cleft surgeons suggest that the Furlow double opposing Z-plasty technique be limited to clefts of the soft palate, the author has used a modification of Furlow's technique for closure of clefts involving the hard palate [39]. Furlow's technique for hard palate closure involves closing the hard palate defect by oral displacement and tenting of the hard palate mucoperiosteal flaps across the cleft, creating a dead space between the hard palate mucosal closure and the bone and nasal mucosal closure (Fig. 17) [4,39,42]. This dead space is believed to fill with hematoma, which organizes into scar tissue [4,39]. Expansion of the hematoma is believed to contribute to fistula formation [4]. The risk for fistula formation with this technique increases with clefts greater than 1 cm in diameter because of excessive tension on the midline area of closure [39]. The author has experienced an unacceptable rate of fistulae at the junction of the hard and soft palates with this technique and currently uses a combination double opposing Z-plasty closure of the soft palate and two-flap closure of the hard palate without fistula formation that is herein described.

Surgical technique. Both the soft and hard palate mucosae are injected with 0.5% lidocaine with 1:200,000 epinephrine. The mucosa is incised along the medial edge of both the hard and soft palate cleft bilaterally. These incisions extend to the premaxilla to repair the alveolar cleft, if present. Early

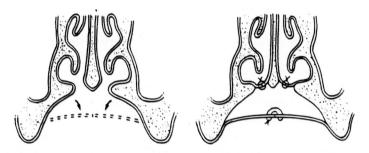

Fig. 17. Position of hard palate oral mucosa relative to nasal mucosa and underlying bone with Furlow hard palate mucosal closure and two-flap hard palate mucosal closure. (*Adapted from* Gage-White L. Furlow palatoplasty: double opposing Z-plasty. Facial Plast Surg 1993;9:181–3; and Nguyen PN, Sullivan PK. Issues and controversies in the management of cleft palate. Clin Plast Surg 1993;20:671–82; with permission.)

gingivoperiosteoplasty, in addition to promoting nasal hygiene and normal speech development, has been shown to result in sufficient alveolar bone development in 25% to 80% of patients to allow the eruption of primary and permanent dentition [41,43]. The technique for repair of the unilateral complete cleft palate is identical for that of repair of the soft palate cleft to the point of transposition of the velar oral mucosal flaps. Before transposition of the soft palate oral mucosal flaps, the repair of the bony palatal cleft is completed.

The nasal closure is performed first by elevating the mucoperiosteum of the nasal floor and vomer. If the cleft is wide, elevation of the nasal floor mucoperiosteum may be carried laterally to the nasal sidewall to allow sufficient medial advancement of the nasal floor mucosa to allow tensionless closure. If the cleft is so wide that there is insufficient nasal floor mucoperiosteum, the vomerine mucoperiosteum is sutured to the ipsilateral palatal shelf bone to close the nasal floor.

The hard palate mucosa is then incised from the maxillary tuberosities and along the base of the alveolar bone to meet the incisions at the cleft edges. Bilateral mucoperiosteal flaps are elevated, with care being taken to preserve the greater palatine vessels. The velar oral mucosal flaps are transposed, and the hard palate oral mucosal flaps are approximated in the midline with interrupted vertical mattress sutures.

Gingivoperiosteoplasty is performed at this point if the cleft extends to the alveolus. The mucosa on both the labial and lingual sides of the alveolus is elevated on both sides of the cleft. Extensive mobilization of the mucosa may be required to achieve tensionless closure. Recruitment of labial mucosa for closure of the alveolar cleft is discouraged because this tethers the lip. The alveolar mucosal flaps are approximated across the cleft. After gingivoperiosteoplasty is completed, the hard palate oral mucosa may be loosely tacked to the alveolar mucosa, or an obturator may be applied for seven to ten days to facilitate adherence of the hard palate mucosa to the palatal bone.

Bilateral complete cleft palate

Although the bilateral complete cleft palate is often wider than the unilateral complete cleft palate, the principles of closure are the same. As described for closure of the unilateral complete cleft palate, the double opposing Z-plasty flaps are designed in the soft palate, and closure of the soft palate nasal mucosa is completed. Bilateral vomer and nasal floor mucoperiosteal flaps are developed. Once the bilateral nasal floor closure is completed, the hard palate oral mucosal flaps are developed. Although the hard palate mucosal flaps may be mobilized completely and tethered only on the greater palatine neurovascular bundles, significant tension may still exist in the midline closure area at the hard palate–soft palate junction. This is because the double opposing Z-plasty closure of the soft palate precludes large back-cuts in the soft palate oral mucosa to preserve the vascularity of the soft palate flaps. In such situations, the author has found it useful to reinforce the palatal mucosal closure by suturing a strip of acellular human dermal matrix (Alloderm Lifecell, Branchburg, New Jersey) to the palatal mucosa in the midline before transposition of the soft palate oral mucosal flaps and closure of the hard palate mucosal flaps. This technique has been found useful in the prevention of fistulae when the palatal cleft is wide and the mucosa of the palatal shelves is limited.

Postoperative care

Patients are observed postoperatively with continuous pulse oximetry for the first 24 to 48 postoperative hours because of the risk for upper airway edema and hemorrhage. A mist tent may be used. Intravenous hydration is maintained and intravenous pain medications, supplemented with acetaminophen suppositories, are administered until the child demonstrates adequate feeding behavior. Arm splints are placed and maintained for the first two postoperative weeks to prevent patient disruption of the palatal repair. Clear liquids are introduced by syringe or cup on the first postoperative day, and nipple feeding is discouraged. A liquid diet is maintained for 1 to 2 weeks. Patients are discharged when oral alimentation is adequate [4].

Complications and their management

Respiratory compromise. Respiratory compromise in the immediate postoperative period can be life threatening and is related to upper airway edema or excessive sedation. This complication is best prevented by close monitoring of patients in a pediatric intensive care unit for the first 24 to 48 hours, and may require intubation. The application of a mist tent postoperatively may decrease upper airway obstruction.

Hemorrhage. Blood loss during cleft palate repair can be significant. This problem can be controlled by injecting the palatine mucosa with an epinephrine-containing local anesthetic before surgery. In addition, neurosurgical patties soaked in 1:200,000 topical epinephrine should be applied to open areas during the procedure. Cauterization should be used conservatively to preserve viability of the mucosal flaps.

Oronasal fistulae. The incidence of palatal fistula formation is reported to be between 3.4% and 29% [4,44]. The success of fistula repair is limited [4]. Previously closed oronasal fistulae tend to reopen during palatal expansion [45]. Fistulae are usually the result of poor tissue quality and excess wound tension. This emphasizes the importance of gentle tissue handling with complete flap mobilization. In addition, the use of postoperative arm splints decreases the risk for wound dehiscence caused by patient manipulation [4].

Long palate. Excessive palatal length has been reported with the double op- posing Z-plasty technique, leading to airway obstruction in neurologically compromised children. The surgeon may consider straight-line repairs in such clinical situations [39].

Secondary correction of cleft-related problems

Velopharyngeal dysfunction

The incidence of velopharyngeal dysfunction varies from study to study and has been reported to be between 20% and 83%. It is believed to depend on the type of palatal repair. Other contributing factors are the extent and width of the cleft, which impact the amount of tissue available for repair; the extent of undermining necessary, which in turn affects scarring; and the length of the native velum. Velopharyngeal dysfunction manifests as in- creased nasality, nasal emission, weakening of pressure consonants, and na- sal reflux [33]. Speech therapy is initiated in the postoperative period and continued until the dysfunction and compensatory misarticulations are cor- rected. Persistent velopharyngeal dysfunction is best addressed surgically with a pharyngeal flap procedure between the ages of 5 and 6 years, but at- tendant risks of this procedure include the development of hyponasal reso- nance and sleep apnea. The placement of a palatal prosthesis is another treatment option, but is often poorly tolerated.

Alveolar bone grafting

Indications for alveolar bone grafting include stabilization of the max- illary arch, provision of bony support to the teeth neighboring the cleft, closure of oronasal fistulae (if present), elevation of the cleft nasal base, and facilitation of orthodontic treatment or placement of titanium im- plants. Secondary alveolar bone grafting is generally preferred to primary grafting at the time of cleft lip or palate repair because of the adverse ef- fects of primary grafting on facial growth [46,47]. Secondary alveolar bone grafting is ideally performed before eruption of the permanent canine tooth and, if possible, before eruption of the lateral incisor. Iliac crest can- cellous bone is the most widely used donor site, but other sites include the tibial shaft, mandibular symphysis, rib, and split calvarial bone [48]. Yen and colleagues [49] reported a novel approach to closure of a large alve- olar cleft that was too large for bone grafting because of soft tissue insuf- ficiency. Orthodontic springs, elastics, and wires were used to transport a posterior segment of bone containing two premolars in a patient with bilateral cleft lip and palate. The authors report that other craniofacial teams are studying distraction methods for closure of large alveolar clefts.

Midfacial hypoplasia

The timing of CP repair at age 9 to 12 months optimizes speech development; however, it is recognized that palatal repairs that denude bone heal with scar contracture resulting in midfacial growth distortion. This midfacial growth retardation results in a prognathic profile (see Fig. 13). As important as the aesthetic consequences of midfacial hypoplasia are its effects on speech. Class III malocclusion can affect production of all the tongue tip and bilabial consonants. Anterior open bite and lateral open bite may result in a lisp. Moreover, a lowered palatal vault, which can occur with some types of hard palate cleft repair, can result in restricted tongue mobility and distortion of the midline palatal groove necessary for production of some sibilant consonants [32,33].

Correction of maxillary hypoplasia and retrusion usually requires transverse maxillary expansion during the period of mixed dentition to correct lingual crossbite deformities and orthognathic surgical correction during the second decade of life. Anterior-inferior maxillary advancement with Le-Fort I osteotomies and rigid fixation is plagued by relapse. The use of postoperative protraction facemasks has been advocated to prevent surgical relapse in cleft lip and palate patients following LeFort I osteotomy [50]. Maxillary distraction osteogenesis is associated with a reduced relapse rate because of its ability to combine new bone deposition with bone remodeling and maxillary advancement. Skeletal-anchored distraction devices are believed to be superior to tooth-borne devices in that the tooth-anchored devices result in greater dental than skeletal movement [51,52].

Secondary septorhinoplasty

Correction of the unilateral cleft nasal deformity remains one of the most challenging aspects of cleft surgical care as evidenced by the number of techniques advocated for this problem. Dutton and Bumsted [53] use a three-tiered approach to correction of the cleft nasal deformity. After performing primary rhinoplasty at the time of lip repair, intermediate rhinoplasty is performed after alveolar bone grafting and closure of the nasolabial fistula. The goal of the intermediate rhinoplasty is to correct any residual lower cartilaginous deformity. An open rhinoplasty approach is used through V-Y advancement flaps from the upper lip to lengthen the columella (a Bardach modification is used for the unilateral cleft lip nasal deformity). A Y-V alar advancement may also be used to narrow the alar base, with fixation of the base to the nasal spine with permanent suture. Delayed rhinoplasty is then performed after puberty to correct any bony dorsal deformity and various causes of nasal obstruction.

In a retrospective review from India, Ahuja [54] described radical correction of the nasal deformity in unilateral cleft lip patients who presented in the second and third decade of life. None of these patients had undergone primary nasal correction, orthodontic management, or alveolar bone grafting before presentation. An open rhinoplasty approach was used. All of the patients were treated with columellar lengthening on the cleft side, submucous resection of the nasal septum with repositioning of the caudal strut, nasal dorsal augmentation, and bone grafting along the pyriform margin, nasal floor, and alveolus. The nasal tip deformity was corrected with interdomal suturing, and the alar cartilages were fixed to the septum and upper lateral cartilages with permanent sutures. Alar base repositioning was performed with a V-Y advancement if excessive flaring of the ala was present. Osteotomies were avoided. Ahuja reported good aesthetic results, while acknowledging some persistent alar base depression, inadequate positioning of the caudal septum, lack of tip definition, nostril asymmetry, and inadequate dorsal augmentation. Although no improvement in occlusion can be obtained with this technique, it is an acceptable corrective measure for patients who present late for correction of cleft nasal deformities and cannot or will not tolerate orthognathic and orthodontic procedures [54].

Future considerations

Care of the patient who has orofacial clefting may change considerably in the not-too-distant future because of advances in the fields of tissue engineering, genetics, and fetal surgery. Ongoing work in molecular developmental biology will increase our understanding of the interactions of the biomolecules involved in craniofacial development and tissue healing. This insight will guide the application of tissue engineering techniques to not only correct the maldevelopment associated with clefting in utero but to facilitate care of the pediatric and adult patient who has cleft lip and palate. For example, the use of bone morphogenetic protein-containing bioresorbable implants has been suggested for repair of alveolar clefting to prevent the morbidity associated with bone graft harvesting [55]. Similarly, as knowledge of the human genome progresses and the various genes involved in orofacial clefting are identified, in utero gene therapy may become feasible as methods of targeted gene delivery are refined. Moreover, a better comprehension of the effects of environmental factors on gene expression may lead to improvements in prenatal care that can significantly reduce the incidence of clefting.

Fetal surgery is an exciting and promising prospect for children who have various craniofacial anomalies. The advantages of fetal surgery include scarless wound healing if performed at midgestation and normalization of facial growth. Fetal cleft lip repair has been demonstrated in various animal models and CP repair has also been demonstrated in utero using a goat model [55–60]. Fetal surgery poses significant risks to the mother and fetus, however, including the risk for premature labor, even with the advent of endoscopic techniques. These risks make in utero cleft repair ethically unjustifiable at this time [55].

References

[1] Strong EB, Buckmiller LM. Management of the cleft palate. Facial Plast Surg Clin North Am 2001;9(1):15–25.
[2] Salyer KE. Excellence in cleft lip and palate treatment. J Craniofac Surg 2001;12(1):2–5.
[3] McInnes RR, Michaud J. Developmental biology: frontiers for clinical genetics. Clin Genet 2002;61:248–56.
[4] Nguyen PN, Sullivan PK. Issues and controversies in the management of cleft palate. Clin Plast Surg 1993;20(4):671–82.
[5] Stanier P, Moore GE. Genetics of cleft lip and palate: syndromic genes contribute to the incidence of non-syndromic clefts. Hum Mol Genet 2004;13(Review Issue Number 1):R73–81.
[6] Jones MC. Facial clefting. Etiology and developmental pathogenesis. Clin Plast Surg 1993; 20(4):599–606.
[7] Kirschner RE, LaRossa D. Cleft lip and palate. Otolaryngol Clin North Am 2000;33(6): 1191–215.
[8] Rollnick BR, Pruzansky S. Genetic services at a center for craniofacial anomalies. Cleft Palate J 1981;18(4):304–13.
[9] Cobourne MT. The complex genetics of cleft lip and palate. Eur J Orthod 2004;26(1):7–16.
[10] Jugessur A, Murray JC. Orofacial clefting: recent insights into a complex trait. Curr Opin Genet Dev 2005;15(3):270–8.
[11] Robin NH, Franklin J, Prucka S, et al. Clefting, amniotic bands, and polydactyly: a distinct phenotype that supports an intrinsic mechanism for amniotic band sequence. Am J Med Genet A 2005;137(3):298–301.
[12] Prescott NJ, Winter RM, Malcolm S. Nonsyndromic cleft lip and palate: complex genetics and environmental effects. Ann Hum Genet 2001;65(6):505–15.
[13] Wong FK, Hägg U. An update on the aetiology of orofacial clefts. Hong Kong Med J 2004; 10(5):331–6.
[14] Kerrigan JJ, Mansell JP, Sengupta A, et al. Palatogenesis and potential mechanisms for clefting. J R Coll Surg Edinb 2000;45(6):351–8.
[15] Spritz RA. The genetics and epigenetics of orofacial clefts. Curr Opin Pediatr 2001;13(6): 556–60.
[16] Moore KL. The branchial apparatus and the head and neck. In: Moore KL, editor. Before we are born: basic embryology and birth defects. 3rd edition. Philadelphia: WB Saunders; 1989. p. 134–58.
[17] Jones KL. Facial defects as major feature. In: Smith's recognizable patterns of human malformation. 5th edition. Philadelphia: WB Saunders; 1997. p. 230–55.
[18] Jones KL. Facial-limb defects as major feature. In: Smith's recognizable patterns of human malformation. 5th edition. Philadelphia: WB Saunders; 1997. p. 256–99.
[19] Trier WC. Repair of unilateral cleft lip: the rotation-advancement operation. Clin Plast Surg 1985;12(4):573–94.
[20] Sykes JM. Management of the cleft lip deformity. Facial Plast Surg Clin North Am 2001; 9(1):37–50.
[21] Elmendorf EN, D'Antonio LL, Hardesty RA. Assessment of the patient with cleft lip and palate: a developmental approach. Clin Plast Surg 1993;20(4):607–21.
[22] Mulliken JB, Pensler JM, Kozakewich HPW. The anatomy of Cupid's bow in normal and cleft lip. Plast Reconstr Surg 1993;92(3):395–403.
[23] Fara M, Chlumska A, Hrivnakova J. Musculis orbicularis oris in incomplete hare lip. Acta Chir Plast (Prague) 1965;7:125–32.
[24] Wilhelmsen HR, Musgrave RH. Complications of cleft lip surgery. Cleft Palate J 1966;3: 223–31.
[25] Cho B. Unilateral complete cleft lip and palate repair using lip adhesion and passive alveolar molding appliance. J Craniofac Surg 2001;12(2):148–56.

[26] Vig KWL, Turvey TA. Orthodontic-surgical interaction in the management of cleft lip and palate. Clin Plast Surg 1985;12(4):735–48.

[27] Witt PD, Hardesty RA. Rotation-advancement repair of the unilateral cleft lip: one center's perspective. Clin Plast Surg 1993;20(4):633–45.

[28] LaRossa D, Donath G. Primary nasoplasty in unilateral and bilateral cleft nasal deformity. Clin Plast Surg 1993;20(4):781–91.

[29] Mulliken JB. Primary repair of bilateral cleft lip and nasal deformity. Plast Reconstr Surg 2001;108(1):181–94.

[30] Mulliken JB, Burvin R, Farkas LG. Repair of bilateral complete cleft lip: intraoperative nasolabial antropometry. Plast Reconstr Surg 2001;107(2):307–14.

[31] Wilson LF. Correction of residual deformities of the lip and nose in repaired clefts of the primary palate (lip and alveolus). Clin Plast Surg 1985;12(4):719–33.

[32] Gibbon FE. Abnormal patterns of tongue-palate contact in the speech of individuals with cleft palate. Clin Linguist Phon 2004;18(4–5):285–311.

[33] Harding A, Grunwell P. Characteristics of cleft palate speech. Eur J Disord Commun 1996; 31(4):331–57.

[34] van Lierde KM, Monstrey S, Bonte K, et al. The long-term speech outcome in Flemish young adults after two different types of palatoplasty. Int J Pediatr Otorhinolaryngol 2004;68: 865–75.

[35] da Silva Filho OG, Calvano F, Assunção AGA, et al. Craniofacial morphology in children with complete unilateral cleft lip and palate: a comparison of two surgical protocols. Angle Orthod 2001;71(4):274–84.

[36] Nandlal B, Utreja A, Tewari A, et al. Effects of variation in the timing of palatal repair on sagittal craniofacial morphology in complete cleft lip and palate children. J Indian Soc Pedod Prev Dent 2000;18(4):153–60.

[37] Rohrich RJ, Love EJ, Byrd HS, et al. Optimal timing of cleft palate closure. Plast Reconstr Surg 2000;106(2):413–21.

[38] Liao Y, Mars M. Hard palate repair timing and facial morphology in unilateral cleft lip and palate: before versus after pubertal peak velocity age. Cleft Palate Craniofac J 2006;43(3): 259–65.

[39] Gage-White L. Furlow palatoplasty: double opposing Z-plasty. Facial Plast Surg 1993;9: 181–3.

[40] Yu CC, Chen PK, Chen YR. Comparison of speech results after Furlow palatoplasty and von Langenbeck palatoplasty in incomplete cleft of the secondary palate. Chang Gung Med J 2001;24(10):628–32.

[41] Anastassov GE, Joos U. Comprehensive management of cleft lip and palate deformities. J Oral Maxillofac Surg 2001;59(9):1062–75.

[42] Furlow LT. Cleft palate repair by double opposing Z-plasty. Plast Reconstr Surg 1986;78: 724–35.

[43] Bitter K. Repair of bilateral cleft lip, alveolus, and palate part 3: follow-up criteria and late results. J Craniomaxillofac Surg 2000;29:49–55.

[44] Wilhelmi BJ, Appelt EA, Hill L, et al. Palatal fistulas: rare with the two-flap palatoplasty repair. Plast Reconstr Surg 2001;107(2):315–8.

[45] Bardach J, Morris HL, Olin WH, et al. Results of multidisciplinary management of bilateral cleft lip and palate at the Iowa Cleft Palate Center. Plast Reconstr Surg 1992;89(3):419–32.

[46] Davis PT, Hochman M, Funcik T. Alveolar cleft bone grafts. Facial Plast Surg 1993;9(3): 232–8.

[47] Newlands LC. Secondary alveolar bone grafting in cleft lip and palate patients. Br J Oral Maxillofac Surg 2000;38(5):488–91.

[48] Kalaaji A, Lilja J, Elander A, et al. Tibia as donor site for alveolar bone grafting in patients with cleft lip and palate: long term experience. Scand J Plast Reconstr Hand Surg 2001;35(1): 35–42.

[49] Yen SL, Gross J, Wang P, et al. Closure of a large alveolar cleft by bony transport of a pos-
     terior segment using orthodontic archwires attached to bone: report of a case. J Oral Max-
     illofac Surg 2001;59(6):688–91.
[50] Gaukroger MJ, Bounds G, Noar JH. The use of a face mask for postoperative retention in
     cleft lip and palate patients. Int J Adult Orthodon Orthognath Surg 2000;15(2):114–8.
[51] Harada K, Baba Y, Ohyama K, et al. Maxillary distraction osteogenesis for cleft lip and pal-
     ate children using an external, adjustable, rigid distraction device: a report of 2 cases. J Oral
     Maxillofac Surg 2001;59(12):1492–6.
[52] Swennen G, Dujardin T, Goris A, et al. Maxillary distraction osteogenesis: a method with
     skeletal anchorage. J Craniofac Surg 2000;11(2):120–7.
[53] Dutton JM, Bumsted RM. Management of the cleft lip nasal deformity. Facial Plast Surg
     Clin North Am 2001;9(1):51–8.
[54] Ahuja RB. Radical correction of secondary nasal deformity in unilateral cleft lip patients
     presenting late. Plast Reconstr Surg 2001;108:1127–35.
[55] Papadopulos NA, Papadopoulos MA, Kovacs L, et al. Foetal surgery and cleft lip and pal-
     ate: current status and new perspectives. Br J Plast Surg 2005;58(5):593–607.
[56] Weinzweig J, Panter KE, Pantaloni M, et al. The fetal cleft palate: II. Scarless healing after in
     utero repair of a congenital model. Plast Reconstr Surg 1999;104(5):1356–64.
[57] Weinzweig J, Panter KE, Spangenberger A, et al. The fetal cleft palate: III. Ultrastructural
     and functional analysis of palatal development following in utero repair of the congenital
     model. Plast Reconstr Surg 2002;109(7):2355–62.
[58] Schutte BC, Murray JC. The many faces and factors of orofacial clefts. Hum Mol Genet
     1999;8(10):1853–9.
[59] Wantia N, Rettinger G. The current understanding of clef lip malformations. Facial Plast
     Surg 2002;18(3):147–53.
[60] Weinberg SM, Neiswanger K, Martin RA, et al. The Pittsburgh oral-facial cleft study: ex-
     panding the cleft phenotype. Background and justification. Cleft Palate Craniofac J 2006;
     43(1):7–20.

ELSEVIER
SAUNDERS

Otolaryngol Clin N Am
40 (2007) 61–80

OTOLARYNGOLOGIC
CLINICS
OF NORTH AMERICA

Microtia and Congenital Aural Atresia

Peggy E. Kelley, MD*, Melissa A. Scholes, MD

*Department of Otolaryngology, University of Colorado Health Sciences Center,
4200 East 9th Avenue, B205, Denver, CO 80220, USA*

Microtia is the abnormal development of the external ear that results in a malformed auricle. The deformity that results can range from mild distortion of the anatomic landmarks to the complete absence of the ear (Figs. 1–3). Congenital aural atresia (CAA), which is commonly associated with microtia, is the failure of the development of the external auditory canal (EAC).

Microtia and CAA are relatively rare deformities; still, an otolaryngologist can expect to be called on to evaluate this defect several times in the average career. Although not every otolaryngologist will perform the complex surgical reconstruction of these malformations, one should be familiar with the etiology, anatomy, medical management, and nonsurgical options available for microtia and CAA. The goal of this article is to provide an overview of these areas, and to give an update of current trends and future directions.

These deformities do not exist independent of other malformations of the auditory system. A discussion of middle and inner ear abnormalities is covered elsewhere in this issue.

Epidemiology and etiology

A number of causes have been implicated in the genesis of microtia, including teratogens (such as vitamin A) [1], vascular insults, and genetic aberrations. Isolated microtia results when the branchial arches develop abnormally. When part of a syndrome, microtia/atresia may be a result of a single gene deletion, or the result of embryopathic development, such as in Goldenhar syndrome. Some auricular deformities are a result of multifactorial insults to the fetus [2]. Microtia and CAA occur in approximately 1

---

* Corresponding author. Department of Otolaryngology, The Children's Hospital, 1056 East 19th Avenue, Denver, CO 80218.

E-mail address: kelley.peggy@tchden.org (P.E. Kelley).

doi:10.1016/j.otc.2006.10.003
oto.theclinics.com

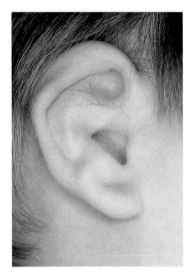

Fig. 1. Atresia without microtia. (*Courtesy of* Glenn Isaacson, MD, Philadelphia, PA.)

in 10,000 to 20,000 births. Both occur more often unilaterally, with a predilection for the right side. Men are affected more than women, at a 2.5:1 ratio. Microtia is commonly associated with CAA, and the degree of auricular malformation usually correlates with the degree of middle ear deformity. However, the incidence of inner ear abnormalities is relatively low in patients who have CAA [3]. Microtia is also associated with other anomalies approximately 50% of the time, especially the facioauriculovertebral

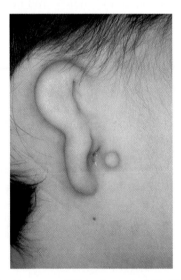

Fig. 2. Microtia. (*Courtesy of* Glenn Isaacson, MD, Philadelphia, PA.)

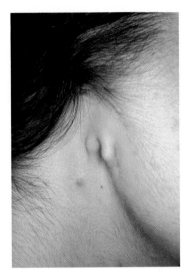

Fig. 3. Severe microtia and atresia. (*Courtesy of* Glenn Isaacson, MD, Philadelphia, PA.)

syndromes. Microtia is seen in higher numbers in Japanese, Hispanic, and Native American populations (particularly the Eskimo and Navajo) [4–6]. Women with four or more pregnancies are at increased risk for having a child with microtia, especially its most severe form, anotia [7]. CAA is more often bony than membranous.

Embryology

During the sixth week of gestation, the external ear begins to develop around the dorsal end of the first branchial cleft. On either side of the cleft lies the first (mandibular) and second (hyoid) branchial arches. The auricle arises from these arches as six small buds of mesenchyme, known traditionally as the six hillocks of His. The mandibular arch gives rise to hillocks 1 through 3, and the hyoid arch gives rise to hillocks 4 through 6 [5,8,9]. Traditionally, it is thought that the derivation of specific auricle components comes from certain hillocks (ie, hillock 1 becomes the tragus, hillocks 2 and 3 form the helix, hillocks 4 and 5 form the antihelix, and hillock 6 forms the lobule). Other theories suggest that the hyoid arch contributes approximately 85% of the auricle, and that most of the central ear is formed from hillocks 4 and 5, whereas the tragus is formed from hillocks 1 through 3. The lobule is the last component of the external ear to develop. The concha is derived from the ectoderm forming the EAC [2,4]. The auricle begins in the anterior neck region, then migrates dorsally and cephalad as the mandible develops during gestational weeks 8 through 12, and lies in its relative adult location by gestational week 20 [10].

During the first and second months' gestation, the external auditory meatus develops from the first branchial groove between the mandibular and hyoid arches. At 4 to 5 weeks' gestation, a solid epithelial nest forms at the meatus, and contacts the endoderm of the first pharyngeal pouch. Mesoderm interrupts the contact between the endoderm and ectoderm. At 8 weeks, the cavum conchae invaginates, forming the primary meatus, which becomes surrounded by cartilage and eventually becomes the fibrocartilaginous portion of the EAC. This groove deepens and grows toward the tympanic cavity and comes into contact with the epithelium of the first pharyngeal pouch. A solid epidermal plug extends from the primary meatus to the primitive tympanic cavity to form the meatal plate (Fig. 4). This plug of tissue recanalizes during the twenty-first week, forming the primitive EAC, and by the twenty-eighth week, only the most medial ectoderm remains, forming the superficial layer of the tympanic membrane (Fig. 5). The ectoderm lines the bony portion of the EAC [5].

Anatomy

The fully formed auricle is a complex, three-dimensional structure with three portions, the helical–antihelical complex, the conchal complex, and the lobule. The elastic cartilage of the auricle is flexible but strong, and is covered loosely with fibrofatty tissue over the margin of the helix and the lobule; adherent skin covers the rest of the cartilaginous framework (Fig. 6) [10].

Ears reach mature size earlier in females than males, at 13 and 15 years, respectively. Normal ear height is between 5.5 and 6.5 cm. The helical rim protrudes from the mastoid surface around 1.5 to 2.0 cm, creating an angle of 15 to 20 degrees [4]. The projection increases from superior to inferior, with the helical rim positioned 10 to 12 mm from the skull, and the lower ear 20 to 22 mm from the skull. The superior edge of the auricle should

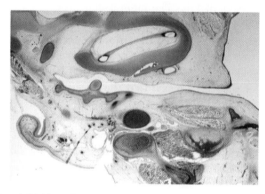

Fig. 4. 12-week fetus initial invagination. (*Courtesy of* Glenn Isaacson, MD, Philadelphia, PA.)

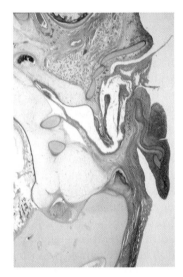

Fig. 5. 18-week fetus recanalization. (*Courtesy of* Glenn Isaacson, MD, Philadelphia, PA.)

be in line with the lateral edge of the eyebrow or the level of the upper eyelid [10]. The ear is inclined posteriorly anywhere from 5 to about 30 degrees along its vertical axis. Classic teaching states that the angle is parallel to the dorsum of the nose, which is not necessarily true, although the two angles are usually within 15 degrees of each other [4,11]. The nose is the more variable angle. With a high nasion, the nose is more upright, but if the

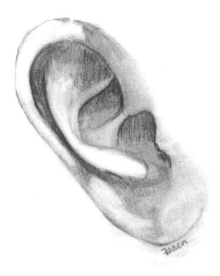

Fig. 6. Fully formed ear with three portions, the helical–antihelical complex, conchal complex, and lobule.

nasion is lower, the radix is flatter and may not be parallel with the axis of the ear (Fig. 7).

The primary blood supply to the auricle is by way of the superficial temporal artery and the posterior auricular artery. Multiple communications between the two arteries allow one of the vessels to supply the ear if necessary. Venous drainage of the ear is by way of the posterior auricular veins that drain into the superficial temporal, external jugular, and retromandibular veins. The great auricular nerve (C3) supplies most of sensation to the external ear, along with small contributions from the lesser occipital nerve (C2,3), auriculotemporal nerve (V3), and cranial nerves VII and X. The ear is attached to the cranium by way of skin, cartilage, and the extrinsic auricular muscles. These extrinsic muscles include the anterior, superior, and posterior suspensory muscles. Intrinsic muscles are present, but play no role in the support or function of the ear [2,10].

The EAC is composed of a lateral cartilaginous (one third) and medial bony (two thirds) canal. The cartilaginous portion is covered with loose skin containing sebaceous glands, ceruminous glands, and hair follicles. The skin overlying the bony canal is thin and tightly adherent. The EAC is curved in a superior and anterior direction [10].

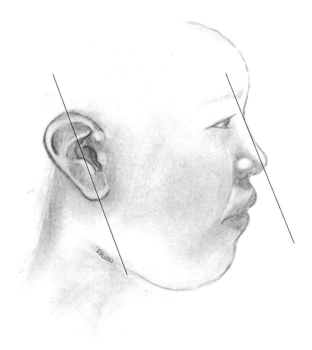

Fig. 7. The angle of the ear is parallel to the dorsum of the nose, usually within 15 degrees of each other.

Initial evaluation

During the initial physical examination, close attention should be paid to the mandible, oral cavity, cervical spine, and eyes, to rule out associated anomalies. Evaluation of the malformed ear should include the quality of the skin, the hairline, and the position of the remnant ear. The integrity of the facial nerve on the malformed side should be assessed because microtia and facial nerve dysfunction are often associated [4,12].

Patients who have unilateral microtia and CAA usually have normal hearing in the contralateral ear [13]. Hearing status, however, is the first thing that should be evaluated in the patient lacking other major developmental anomalies. Sensorineural, conductive, and mixed losses can be seen in the microtic/atretic ear [4,14] Conductive hearing loss represents 80% to 90% of the loss in these patients; however, approximately 10% to 15% will have a sensorineural hearing loss (SNHL) that must be addressed [2]. Patients who have Goldenhar syndrome may have hearing loss in the nonmicrotic ear that is conductive or sensorineural [15]. The threshold of conductive loss on the affected side is expected to be between 40 and 60 dB [13]. In most states, universal newborn hearing screening is mandatory. If the nonmicrotic ear passes the newborn hearing screen, additional testing can be delayed until age 6 to 7 months because hearing is adequate for the acquisition of speech and language. Any hearing concerns before this time require that diagnostic auditory brainstem response testing be performed to be sure at least one ear has normal hearing. In patients who have one malformed ear, careful attention is paid to the normal ear. Any threat to a normal hearing ear should be dealt with promptly. Middle ear effusions should be treated aggressively [2,16].

In cases of bilateral atresia, bilateral bone conduction hearing aids should be placed [5]. Traditionally, hearing amplification is not required in unilateral atresia. However, it is now well-established that binaural hearing is superior to monaural in terms of sound localization and speech perception. Children with a unilateral hearing loss are at a greater risk of developing delayed language development and attention deficit disorders, and of performing poorly in school. The plasticity of the developing auditory system benefits from binaural stimulation, which has led to a push toward improving hearing in patients who have unilateral deficits as well, by way of a surgical correction of CAA (after microtia repair) or by placement of a hearing amplification device [2,12]. Current Food and Drug Administration indications for bone-anchored amplification include age more than 5 years. Typically, microtia repair is performed no earlier than age 6 years, so that CAA drill-out is not before age 7 years. It is unknown if opening the ear at this later time allows for binaural brain development, or if a sensitive period in development has already passed.

CT can be performed to assess middle and inner ear anomalies. Some recommend obtaining this information as early as possible, when the child is several months old, because cholesteatoma is estimated to be present in 4% to 7% of atretic ears and should be ruled out. However, a congenital cholesteatoma often requires several years to grow enough to be evident or problematic, so the CT scan may be delayed until an age where sedation is not required, usually at age 4. If obtained in the newborn period, CT will need to be repeated later if a drill-out procedure for CAA is contemplated, because the temporal bone matures and changes in the first years of life. When obtained at the approximate age of 4, only one CT scan is required. The presence of cholesteatoma or otitis media that is refractory to antibiotics is an indication for surgery, even if a good hearing result is not anticipated [5].

Congenital ear malformations are not detected readily before birth, and may cause psychosocial trauma to the parents and family [3]. Counseling the family members is an important part of the management of these conditions. The expectations of the parents and the reality of the problem may not coincide. It is important to communicate to the family that although microtia reconstruction will improve the appearance of the auricle, the ear may never look normal. Likewise, operations to improve hearing loss caused by CAA rarely achieve normal hearing. It is important that children with these malformations are evaluated early to rule out associated problems, evaluate hearing status, and develop a plan of management.

History of ear reconstruction

Reports of attempted ear reconstruction date as far back as the 1500s. More often than not, these early attempts resulted in failure. The use of autogenous cartilage and improved understanding of reconstructive methods ushered in a new era in the correction of these deformities in the 1930s. Tanzer is credited as the father of modern auricular reconstruction based on an autologous cartilage graft framework placed beneath the skin. Others have refined these techniques to the current practice standards [2,14].

Classification schemes

Any discussion of microtia usually begins with classifying the severity of the irregularity by a grading system. Several grading systems exist and have been modified over the years. All of the classification schemes classify a normal or near-normal auricle as Grade I, with increasing grades signifying increasing deformity. Grade III/IV usually signifies a classic "peanut ear" or complete anotia [8].

The first classification system for microtia was developed by Marx in 1926 [17]. It was later amended by Jarhsdoerfer and Aguilar in 1988 [18]. Aguilar further refined the system, which took into account only malformations of the auricle [19]. Microtia accompanied by atresia is harder to put into simple categories, but several grading strategies exist. Altmann (1955) [20], Lapchenko (1967) [21], and Gill (1969) [22] all developed scales looking at not only the external anatomy but also the status of the rest of the temporal bone. In 1974, Rogers proposed a four-part classification [23]. Tanzer's 1977 publication proposed a clinical classification of auricular abnormalities that is used widely [24]. In 1988, Weerda compiled all the classification systems into one scheme that includes clinical grading and basic management principles (Box 1) [8,14]. As classification systems vary over time and between users, the deformity may best be recorded in the physical examination with a description of how it varies from normal. Classification can then be assigned later.

Two popular grading classifications for CAA are the De la Cruz classification and the Jahrsdorfer grading system. The De la Cruz classification divides malformations into minor and major categories. Ears with minor abnormalities are better surgical candidates, whereas those with major abnormalities may be better served by a hearing aid. The Jahrsdorfer grading system assigns points to certain CT characteristics, with a higher score determining a better surgical candidate (Tables 1 and 2) [5].

Microtia repair

Microtia deformities range from mild to severe, as seen with the grading schemes in Box 1 and Table 2. For mild, or type I, microtia, basic reconstructive techniques for surgical correction apply. Various techniques of cartilage reshaping and sculpturing have been described for moderate deformities. In this article, the authors concentrate on the surgical techniques involved in the repair of severe microtia and anotia.

Microtia repair using autogenous cartilage is the gold standard of surgical reconstruction. As mentioned earlier, this technique was refined by Tanzer and consists of a multistage operative technique. The stages range in number from two to four, with about 3 months' separation between stages. This method remains the standard because of the high quality and reproducibility of the repair, and continued patient satisfaction [11]. It is a very challenging practice, however, and various techniques have emerged that are surgeon specific. The senior author of this article follows the technique of Brent with minor modifications, as described in the following paragraphs [25].

The first stage consists of designing a template of the normal ear to use as a guide. In patients who have low-lying hairlines, a smaller ear may be designed to avoid a hair-bearing ear. The template is used to estimate the correct graft position. The usual landmarks include the upper eyelid, nose, and lobule, if present. If hemifacial microsomia is present, the superior margin of the contralateral ear is used [14,16].

In the first stage, cartilage is harvested from the contralateral sixth through eighth ribs. Harvesting from the contralateral side provides a better curvature to the graft (Fig. 8). The base of the new ear is formed from the synchondrosis of the sixth and seventh rib. The floating eighth rib is used to

Box 1. Weerda's combined classification of auricular defects, including surgical recommendations

First-degree dysplasia. Average definition: most structures of a normal auricle are recognizable (minor deformities). Surgical definition: Reconstruction does not require the use of additional skin or cartilage.
a. Microtia
b. Protruding ear (synonyms: prominent ear, bat ear)
c. Cryptotia (synonyms: pocket ear, group IV B (Tanzer))
d. Absence of upper helix
e. Small deformities: absence of the tragus, satyr ear, Darwinian tubercle, additional folds (Stahl ear)
f. Colobomata (synonyms: clefts, transverse coloboma)
g. Lobule deformities (pixed lobule, macrolobule, absence of lobule, lobule colobamata (bifid lobule))
h. Cup ear deformities
   Type I: cupped upper portion of the helix, hypertrophic concha, reduced height (synonyms: lidding helix, constricted helix, group IV A (Tanzer), lop ear
   Type II: more severe lopping of the upper pole of the ear; rib cartilage is used as support when a short ear must be expanded or the auricular cartilage is limp

Second-degree dysplasia. Average definition: some structures of a normal auricle are recognizable. Surgical definition: partial reconstruction requires the use of some additional skin and cartilage. Synonym: Second-degree microtia (Marx)
a. Cup ear deformity, type III: the severe sup ear deformity is mal formed in all dimensions (synonyms: cockleshell ear, constricted helix, group IV (Tanzer), snail-shell ear)
b. Mini-ear

Third degree dysplasia: Average definition: none of the structures of a normal ear is recognizable. Surgical definition: total reconstruction requires the use of skin and large amounts of cartilage. Synonyms: complete hypoplasia group II, peanut ear, third-degree microtia (Marx); normally concomitant congenital atresia is found
a. Unilateral: one ear is normal; no middle ear reconstruction is performed on any child, auricle reconstruction is begun at age 5 or 6 years
b. Bilateral: bone-conduction hearing aid before the first birthday; middle ear surgery at age 4 years without transposition of the vestige; bilateral reconstruction of the auricle at age 5 or 6 years

Anotia

Table 1
De la Cruz classification of congenital aural atresia

Minor malformations	Major malformations
Normal mastoid pneumatization	Poor pneumatization
Normal oval window/footplate	Abnormal or absent oval window/footplate
Reasonable facial nerve–footplate relationship	Abnormal course of the facial nerve
Normal inner ear	Abnormalities of the inner ear

make a helical framework, which is then attached to the base. At times, an extra piece of cartilage is harvested and banked to use for augmentation of the graft's projection. The cartilage scaffold is then placed in a subcutaneous pocket in the proposed auricular area. Care is taken to preserve subdermal vasculature and to elevate enough tissue so as not to put too much pressure on the fragile graft. The lobule is not transposed as in Tanzer's technique. Suction drains are placed, and kept on continuous suction to ensure the skin adheres to the graft to provide adequate molding and contour [11,14,16].

During the second stage, the lobule is transposed into adequate position. Brent believes it is safer and easier to position the remnant this way [25]. This stage is sometimes combined with the third stage, in which the auricular framework is released from the surrounding tissue (Fig. 9). The graft is released by incising the skin several millimeters away from the rim of the graft. Dissection is continued over the posterior surface of the graft until adequate projection is obtained. It is here that the banked piece of cartilage is used to elevate the graft. After positioning the new auricle, the retroauricular scalp is advanced forward. A skin graft is then used to cover the medial

Table 2
Jahrsdoerfer grading system of candidacy for atresiaplasty

Parameter	Points
Stapes present	2
Oval window open	1
Middle ear space	1
Facial nerve normal	1
Malleus–incus complex present	1
Mastoid well-pneumatized	1
Incus–stapes connection	1
Round window normal	1
Appearance of external ear	1

Rating	Type of candidate
10	Excellent
9	Very good
8	Good
7	Fair
6	Marginal
≤ 5	Poor

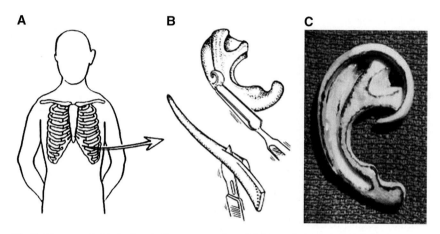

Fig. 8. Framework fabrication in the young patient. (*A*) To optimize natural configuration, rib cartilage is harvested from the chest opposite to the side of the ear defect. (*B*) The framework is sculpted in two pieces: the ear's main body is carved from synchondrotic cartilage block, and the helix is created by thinning the floating cartilage on the outer, convex surface to warp it into a favorable curve. (*C*) The completed framework. The helix has been affixed to the main block with 4 to 5 sutures of 4-0 clear nylon, with the knots placed on the frame's undersurface. (*From* Brent B. Microtia repair with rib cartilage grafts. A review of personal experience with 1000 cases. Clin Plastic Surg 2002;29:257–271.)

portion of the graft and the immediate postauricular area. Split thickness [11,14,16] and full thickness skin grafts have been described [25].

The fourth stage involves reconstructing the tragus, creating a concha, and making adjustments for symmetry. Sometimes a piece of cartilage is used from the conchal area of the contralateral ear for tragus reconstruction, which allows some manipulation of the normal ear to help with symmetry. Some opponents of this method disapprove of taking material from the "normal ear." Alternatively, an additional piece of rib can be harvested during stage one to create an antitragus–tragus unit that is attached to the base (Fig. 10) [11,14,16].

Another popular technique is the two-stage method developed by Nagata [26], which involves constructing the auricular framework from the sixth through ninth ribs, including the tragus, which is assembled using stainless-steel sutures. These sutures have been associated with extrusion. Obviously, the amount of cartilage harvested is significant and could lead to a chest-wall deformity. Thus, Nagata leaves the perichondrium in situ to stimulate cartilage growth. The framework is placed and the lobule remnant is transposed. The posterior skin of the lobule is used to cover the tragus and conchal parts of the graft. Six months later, the second stage of reconstruction is performed and the graft is released. Another rib graft from the fifth rib is used to elevate the framework, requiring another chest-wall incision. A split-thickness skin graft is then used to cover the posterior portion of the graft [11,14,26].

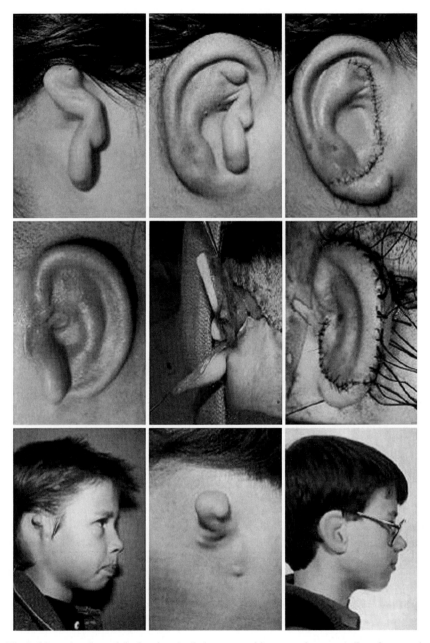

Fig. 9. Managing the earlobe in microtia. Lobe transposition secondary to cartilage framework stage (*top*). Lobe transposition combined with elevation procedure (*middle*), which was safe because the skin-bridge above the short lobule carries circulation across to the auricle. Microtia with absent lobule vestige (*bottom*). The lobe is created by first defining it in the rib carving, then further delineating it when the ear is elevated with skin graft. (*From* Brent B. Microtia repair with rib cartilage grafts. A review of personal experience with 1000 cases. Clin Plastic Surg 2002;29:257–71.)

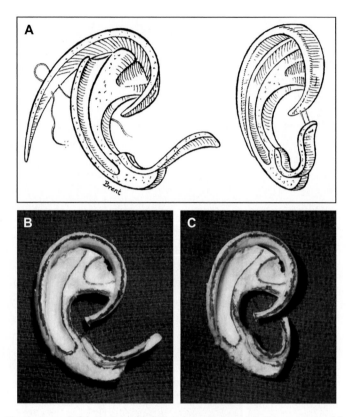

Fig. 10. Ear framework fabrication with integral tragal strut. (*A*) Construction of frame. The floating cartilage creates helix, and second strut is arched around to form antitragus, intertragal notch and tragus. This arch is completed when the tip of the strut is affixed to the crus helix of the main frame with a horizontal mattress suture of clear nylon. (*B*) and (*C*) Actual framework fabrication with patient's rib cartilage. (*From* Brent B. Microtia repair with rib cartilage grafts. A review of personal experience with 1000 cases. Clin Plastic Surg 2002;29:257–71.)

The optimal age to perform microtia repair is a matter of debate. Some of the influencing factors include maturity of the ear, available rib cartilage, and psychosocial issues. The usual age is between 6 and 8 years. The auricle reaches 95% of its adult size at age 6 years. Brent usually begins repair at age 6 in girls, and, in boys, recommends waiting longer, up to age 10, when they comply more easily with postoperative instructions. Nagata waits until the patient is 10 years old or the chest circumference is 60 cm, which is required secondary to the amount of rib cartilage necessary in his repair technique [11,14].

Complications of microtia repair

When the complexity of the reconstruction is reviewed, one realizes that even small complications can lead to loss of the flap or graft if care is not taken. A small hematoma or vascular injury can cause a portion of the flap to necrose. If a small part (1–2 mm) of the graft becomes exposed but the perichondrium is intact, oral antibiotic therapy with *Staphylococcal* and *Pseudomonas* coverage should begin. Moist coverage of the cartilage with stringent dressing management should be instituted. Larger defects may require coverage with a local flap, such as a temporoparietal-fascial flap. After flap coverage, long-term antibiotic administration in necessary to avoid the spread of infection and absorption of the graft [4].

Minor cosmetic complications can include poor positioning, scar contracture and hypertrophy, and poor contouring of landmarks. Generally, all will improve with time. Minor scar revisions can be performed after the healing phase is complete [4].

Acute pneumothorax and atelectasis can develop from the harvesting of rib cartilage. Delayed complications of rib harvest include chest-wall deformity and scarring. To avoid complications from pneumothorax, some surgeons advocate the use of chest tubes in the immediate postoperative period after rib harvest. Ohara and colleagues [27] reported a decrease of chest-wall deformity if the patient is older than 10 years at harvest, compared with children younger than 10 (20% and 64%, respectively). However, this age criterion is less well accepted in the western world, where social and peer stresses play a more prominent role in surgical decision making [14].

Congenital aural atresia repair

Repair of an atretic ear canal depends on the likelihood of yielding serviceable hearing [28]. Using classification schemes such as those created by De la Cruz and Jahrsdoerfer helps decide which patient is a good candidate for atresiaplasty. Temporal bone anatomy is reviewed, along with any evidence of other congenital abnormalities [29]. Children with CAA associated with other syndromes (Goldenhar, Treacher-Collins, Crouzon, and so forth) usually are not candidates for surgical atresiaplasty and should be considered for an implantable hearing aid [5].

CAA repair follows microtia repair by 2 months to preserve the vascular supply to the skin and subcutaneous tissues [30]. In patients who have binaural microtia and CAA, this is often done at 6 years of age. For patients who have unilateral atresia, the CAA repair may be delayed until the patient can understand fully the risks of surgery. However, if the mastoid and middle ear spaces are well-pneumatized and normal facial nerve function and ossicles exist, caregivers may elect to go forward with a surgery at a younger age, given the decreased surgical complication risk [5].

A high-resolution CT scan of the temporal bone should be obtained to evaluate the anatomy. The mastoid should be evaluated carefully because the canal is created at the expense of the mastoid. The most important factors for surgical planning include the status of the inner ear, the temporal bone pneumatization, the course of the facial nerve, the presence of the oval window and footplate, and the presence of cholesteatoma. The thickness of the bony plate and the soft tissue components are also evaluated [5].

The three approaches for CAA repair are mastoid, anterior, and modified anterior. The mastoid approach involves drilling out the mastoid and identifying the sinodural angle, which is often difficult because of the distorted anatomy and the risk of damage to the facial nerve, vestibular system, and other structures. The anterior approach is the technique most often used (see later discussion). The modified anterior approach is a variation of the anterior method first described by Murakami and Quatela [4].

According to the anterior method, a postauricular incision is made and the subcutaneous tissue and periosteum are raised anteriorly to the glenoid fossa. If any tympanic bone is present, the drilling is started at the cribriform area. If no tympanic bone is present, the drilling begins at the temporal line just posterior to the glenoid fossa. Drilling continues anteriorly and medially until the epitympanum is entered. The most common associated anomaly of the middle ear space is a fused malleal-incudal joint, whereas the stapes is often normal. The atretic bone is removed carefully, uncovering the ossicles. The facial nerve is always medial to the ossicular mass, but must be avoided in the posterior-inferior middle ear space. Drilling is continued until the new canal is about 10 mm in size. Ossicular reconstruction takes place either with the patient's native ossicles (preferred) or a prosthesis, as necessary. A tympanic membrane is then created using temporalis fascia. A split-thickness skin graft is used to line the new EAC. Finally, a meatoplasty is created to augment the opening, and a large ear wick is inserted to help stent the canal. Reduction in diameter of the new canal by approximately 30% is normal postoperatively [5].

Complications of congenital aural atresia repair

Complications of CAA repair include lateralization of the tympanic membrane graft (22%–28%), stenosis of the canal (8%), temporomandibular joint pain and trauma (2%), facial nerve damage (1%), and SNHL (2%–5%). Lateralization of the graft is avoided by using gelfoam packing to stabilize it during the healing phase. The patient and surgeon must take meticulous care of the canal to avoid stenosis, including regular examinations and debridements, and prompt treatment of any infections. High-frequency SNHL may occur from acoustic drill trauma. Finally, facial nerve monitoring is used because normal anatomic landmarks are often missing [5].

Alternative and adjunctive procedures

Prosthetic devices

New technologic advancements have made prosthetic devices an acceptable alternative to surgery. These devices do require a procedure to place anchors, but the multiple operative stages of an autogenous repair are avoided [14]. Although prosthetics have become more tolerable, they do require daily cleaning and upkeep and may become dislodged. They often have to be replaced every 4 to 5 years [8]. Besides patient preference, some indications for prosthetic reconstruction include failed autogenous construction, severe skeletal and soft-tissue hypoplasia, keloid formation, and an unfavorable hairline [31]. Physicians who treat patients who have microtia should be familiar with prostheticians in their area and should readily refer those patients who may desire or require this method of reconstruction.

Alloplastic framework

The morbidity associated with rib harvest for microtia is significant, and includes scarring, deformity, risk of pneumothorax, and postoperative pain [11]. Frameworks made from alloplastic materials would avoid these problems, but no perfect substance yet exists for this use. The use of silicone implants were introduced in the 1960s and 1970s by Cronin [32] and Ohmori [33]. However, long-term follow-up demonstrated problems with flap erosion and implant extrusion [2]. More recently, porous polyethylene frameworks have been used (Medpore, Porex Surgical, Inc., Noonan, Georgia). This material has low tissue reactivity and allows ingrowth, which improves stabilization. Extrusion of porous polyethylene has been reported, but covering the framework with fascia seems to reduce this complication. Such reconstructions remain very delicate and do not tolerate trauma from sports or direct contact. This material should be considered carefully before being used in a microtia reconstruction [11].

Tissue expansion

The use of tissue expanders before implantation of a microtia framework can avoid the use of skin grafts and may reduce the number of surgical procedures, according to advocates of this technique. With the use of expanders, Hata and Umeda [34] reconstructed the auricle in a single stage. They reported superior skin texture and match, and preservation of innervation to the skin. Park and Chi [11] describe a two-flap method whereby the skin and fascial layers are expanded. These layers are split and the microtia graft is sandwiched between the layers. A skin graft is then placed over the fascial layer. Opponents of tissue expansion state that it is painful, and young children are not always able to tolerate it. Tissue expansion also requires a trip to the operating room and may not reduce the number of surgical procedures. Lastly, some say the skin is too thick owing to the formation of a fibrous capsule around the expander, which can produce poor contouring results [11,12].

Tissue engineering

Ideally, an autogenous auricular framework made from a few cells would be the graft of choice for microtia [35]. Experts in tissue engineering have tried to create just that. Scientists have been able to grow an auricular framework using a biodegradable scaffold implanted with bovine chondrocytes [36]. This framework was implanted into an athymic mouse and an ear-shaped piece of cartilage was produced [11]. Limitations of this method include the difficulty of producing an acceptable match consistently and the fragility of the framework. Also, a large number of chondrocytes must be produced, leading to a lengthy amount of time to grow a framework [11]. More recently, Kamil and colleagues have grown cartilage in a gold framework [36]. Current work is focused on getting cells into alternating life cycles so that normal cell maintenance is possible. To date, gold model ears have cells in the same life cycle stage.

Other advances include the use of a three-dimensional model of a patient's normal ear intraoperatively for accurate assessment as a guide for the graft structure. Three-dimensional modeling of a patient's costal cartilage can also be done using ultrasound techniques. Use of a model allows preoperative planning and design of a graft that can help reduce operating time and the amount of cartilage harvested [11,14].

Summary

Microtia and CAA are congenital anomalies that are so common that every otolaryngologist should be familiar with the initial evaluation and care of the patient. Once associated anomalies have been found and addressed, or ruled out, hearing is assessed and habilitated, as needed. When one ear hears normally, speech and language development should be normal. The normally hearing ear is safeguarded. The gross and fine motor development of the baby or child are not expected to be affected in isolated cases of microtia and CAA. Balance is normal.

Current technologies allow for reconstruction or habilitation of the microtic ear when the child is several years of age. The hope is that tissue engineering can eliminate donor site morbidity, and that temporary prosthetic ears will be unnecessary. Aural atresia work continues to be very dependent on the patient anatomy and the need or desire for better hearing in the affected ear.

References

[1] Shaw GM, Carmichael SL, Kaidarova Z, et al. Epidemiologic characteristics of anotia and microtia in California. Birth Defects Res A Clin Mol Teratol 2004;70(7):474–5.

[2] Walton RL, Beahm EK. Auricular reconstruction for microtia: part I. Anatomy, embryology, and clinical evaluation. Plast Reconstr Surg 2002;109(7):2473–82.

[3] Murphy TP, Burstein F, Cohen S. Management of congenital atresia of the external auditory canal. Otolaryngol Head Neck Surg 1997;116(6 Pt 1):580–4.

[4] Murakami CS, Quatela VC, et al. Reconstruction surgery of the ear: microtia reconstruction. In: Cummings CW, Flint PW, Harker LA, et al, editors. Otolaryngology head and neck surgery. 4th edition. Philadelphia: Mosby; 2004. p. 4422–8.

[5] De la Cruz A, Hansen MR. Reconstruction surgery of the ear: auditory canal and tympanum. In: Cummings CW, Flint PW, Harker LA, et al, editors. Otolaryngology head and neck surgery. 4th edition. Philadelphia: Mosby; 2004. p. 4439–44.

[6] Nelson SM, Berry RI. Ear disease and hearing loss among Navajo children—a mass survey. Laryngoscope 1984;94(3):316–23.

[7] Harris J, Kallen B, Robert E. The epidemiology of anotia and microtia. J Med Genet 1996; 33:809–13.

[8] Cunningham MJ, Aguilar E. Congenital auricular malformation. In: Bailey BJ, Johnson JT, Newlands SD, et al, editors. Otolaryngology head and neck surgery. 4th edition. Philadelphia: Lippincott, Williams and Wilkins; 2006. p. 2691–700.

[9] Lee KJ. Essentials of otolaryngology. 5th edition. 2003. McGraw-Hill.

[10] Zim SA. Microtia reconstruction, an update. Curr Opin Otolaryngol Head Neck Surg 2003; 11(4):275–81.

[11] Park S, Chi D. External ear, aural atresia. Available at: www.emedicine.com. 2005. Accessed October 1, 2006.

[12] Brent B. The team approach to treating the microtia atresia patient. Otolaryngol Clin North Am 2000;33(6):1353–65.

[13] Walton RL, Beahm EK. Auricular reconstruction for microtia: part II. Surgical techniques. Plast Reconstr Surg 2002;110(1):234–49.

[14] Weerda H. Classification of congenital deformities of the auricle. Facial Plast Surg 1988;5: 385.

[15] Scholtz AW, Fish JH III, Kammen-Jolly K, et al. Goldenhar's syndrome: congenital hearing deficit of conductive or sensorineural origin? Temporal bone histopathologic study. Otol Neurotol 2001;22(4):501–5.

[16] Eavey RD, Ryan DP. Refinements in pediatric microtia reconstruction. Arch Otolaryngol Head Neck Surg 1996;122(6):617–20.

[17] Marx H. Die Missblidungen des Ohres. In: Henke F, Lubarsh D, editors. Handbuch der Spez Path Anatomie Histologie. Berlin, Germany: Springer; 1926. p. 620–5.

[18] Aguilar E, Jahrsdoerfer R. The surgical repair of congenital microtia and atresia. Otolaryngol Head Neck Surg 1988;98(6):600–6.

[19] Aguilar E. Auricular reconstruction of congenital microtia (grade III). Laryngoscope 1996; 106(12 Pt 2 Suppl 82):1–26.

[20] Altmann F. Congenital atresia of the ear in men and animals. Ann Otol Rhinol Laryngol 1955;64(3):824–58.

[21] Lapchenko S. On surgery for improving hearing in congenital atresia of the external and middle ear. Vestn Otorinolaringol 1967;29(2):91–4.

[22] Gill NW. Congenital atresia of the ear. A review of the surgical findings in 83 cases. J Laryngol Otol 1969;83:551–87.

[23] Rogers B. Anatomy, embryology, and classification of auricular deformities. In: Tanzer R, Edgerton M, editors. Symposium on reconstruction of the auricle, Vol 10. St. Louis: CV Mosby; 1974. p. 3–11.

[24] Tanzer RC. Congenital deformities of the auricle. In: Converse JM, editor. Reconstructive plastic surgery. 2nd ed. Vol 3. Philadelphia: WB Saunders; 1977. p. 1671–719.

[25] Brent B. The correction of microtia with autogenous cartilage grafts I: the classic deformity. Plast Reconstr Surg 1980;66(1):1–12.

[26] Nagata S. A new method of total reconstruction of the auricle for microtia. Plast Reconstr Surg 1993;92(2):187–201.

[27] Ohara K, Nakamura K, Ohta E. Chest wall deformities and thoracic scoliosis after cartilage graft harvesting. Plast Reconstr Surg 1997;99(4):1030–6.

[28] Lambert PR, Dodson EE. Congenital malformations of the external auditory canal. Otolaryngol Clin North Am 1996;29:741–60.

[29] Ishimoto S, Ito K, Yamosoba T, et al. Correlation between microtia and temporal bone malformation evaluated using grading systems. Arch Otolaryngol Head Neck Surg 2005;131(4): 326–9.

[30] Siegert R. Combined reconstruction of congenital auricular atresia and severe microtia. Laryngoscope 2003;113(11):2021–7.

[31] Thorne CH, Brecht LE, Bradley JP, et al. Auricular reconstruction: indications for autogenous and prosthetic techniques. Plast Reconstr Surg 2001;107:1241–52.

[32] Cronin T. Use of silastic frame for total and subtotal reconstruction of the external ear: preliminary report. Plast Reconstr Surg 1966;37(5):399–405.

[33] Ohmori S. Reconstruction of microtia using the Silastic frame. Clin Plast Surg 1978;5(3): 379–87.

[34] Hata Y, Umeda T. Reconstruction of congenital microtia by using a tissue expander. J Med Dent Sci 2000;47:105–16.

[35] Kamil SH, Vacanti MP, Vancanti CA, et al. Microtia chondrocytes as a donor source for tissue-engineered cartilage. Laryngoscope 2004;114(12):2187–90.

[36] Kamil SH, Vancanti MP, Aminuddin BS, et al. Tissue engineering of a human sized and shaped auricle using a mold. Laryngoscope 2004;114(5):867–70.

ELSEVIER
SAUNDERS

Otolaryngol Clin N Am
40 (2007) 81–96

OTOLARYNGOLOGIC
CLINICS
OF NORTH AMERICA

Anomalies of the Middle and Inner Ear

Kimsey Rodriguez, MD[a], Rahul K. Shah, MD[b],
Margaret Kenna, MD, MPH[c,d,*]

[a]*Department of Otolaryngology–Head and Neck Surgery, Tulane University School
of Medicine, New Orleans, LA, USA*
[b]*Division of Otolaryngology, George Washington University School of Medicine,
Children's National Medical Center, Washington, DC, USA*
[c]*Department of Otology and Laryngology, Harvard Medical School, Massachusetts Eye
and Ear Infirmary, 243 Charles Street, Boston, MA 02114, USA*
[d]*Department of Otolaryngology and Communication Disorders, Children's Hospital Boston,
300 Longwood Avenue, LO-367, Boston, MA 02115, USA*

Middle ear development

The external auditory canal develops from the first branchial groove, between the mandibular and hyoid arches (the first and second branchial arches, respectively). The tympanic ring develops from contact between the ectoderm of the first branchial groove and the first pharyngeal pouch. This contact point is interrupted by mesodermal growth (neural crest mesenchyme) at 8 weeks' gestation. This mesenchyme thins to form the fibrous layer of the tympanic membrane. Thus, the tympanic membrane develops from all three embryologic layers, with ectoderm forming the lateral aspect, mesoderm forming the middle layer, and endoderm from the pharyngeal pouch forming the middle layer. The complete tympanic membrane fuses with the tympanic ring during gestational weeks 9 to 16, with ossification of the tympanic ring occurring after birth [1–3].

At week 3 of gestation, the middle ear forms from the tubotympanic recess. The tubotympanic recess develops from expansion of the first and possibly a small contribution from the second pharyngeal pouch. The tubotympanic recess becomes constricted by the second branchial arch during week 7, resulting in formation of the eustachian tube medially and the tympanic cavity laterally. The middle ear develops from the terminal end of the first pharyngeal pouch, which divides into four sacci representing distinct

* Corresponding author. Department of Pediatric Otolaryngology, Children's Hospital, 300 Longwood Avenue, LO-367, Boston, MA 02115.
E-mail address: margaret.kenna@children.harvard.edu (M. Kenna).

anatomic areas by the time of complete development. The saccus anticus (anterior pouch of Tröltsch), the saccus medius (epitympanum and petrous area), the saccus superior (posterior pouch of Tröltsch, inferior incudal space, and part of the mastoid), and saccus posterior (the round window, the oval window, and the sinus tympani) develop from the terminal end of the first pharyngeal pouch and expand to pneumatize the middle ear. Expansion of the sacci covers the ossicles and lines the tympanic and mastoid cavities. Extension of the tympanic cavity at 18 weeks' gestation leads to formation of the epitympanum.

Ossicular development

The ossicles, muscles, and tendons of the middle ear are formed from the mesenchyme of the middle ear and are covered by the epithelial lining from the first pharyngeal pouch. Blood vessels run under the epithelial lining, tethering structures in a mesenteric fashion. The tensor tympani muscle and tendon are derived from the first branchial arch and thus innervated by the mandibular branch of the trigeminal nerve. The stapedius muscle is derived from the second branchial arch mesoderm and innervated by the seventh cranial nerve (Fig. 1).

Ossicular development starts at the fourth to sixth week as neural crest mesenchyme from the first and second branchial arches becomes further divided by the seventh cranial nerve. Differentiation of the neural crest mesenchymal tissue within the tympanic cavity results in formation of the individual ossicles. The head of the malleus and short crus and body of the incus are derived from the mesenchyme of the first branchial arch (mandibular arch). The manubrium of the malleus; long process of the incus; stapes head, neck, and crura; and the tympanic surface of the footplate are derived from the second branchial arch (hyoid arch). The medial stapes

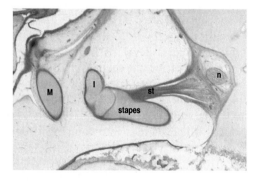

Fig. 1. Photomicrograph of fetal middle ear at 11 weeks' gestation. The future ossicles are composed of cartilage. This cartilage will be replaced by endochondral bone formation except at the articular surfaces. I, incus; M, malleus; n, facial nerve just below the pyramidal eminence; st, stapedial tendon. (*Courtesy of* Glenn Isaacson, MD, Philadelphia, PA.)

footplate and annular stapedial ligament are derived from the otic capsule. The bony otic capsule is adult size by 22 weeks' gestation.

At 6 weeks' gestation, the neural crest mesenchyme forms cartilaginous models of the ossicles, which subsequently grow to adult size by 15 to 18 weeks and completely ossify by 30 weeks. The incus and malleus, previously one collection of cells, separate with formation of the malleoincudal joint at 8 to 9 weeks. Mesenchymal resorption results in the ossicles being free, with the endodermal epithelium tethering the ossicles to the tympanic cavity in a mesentery-like fashion. The stapes ring forms around the transient stapedial artery at 5 to 6 weeks, followed by appearance of the otic capsule mesenchyme. The shape of the stapes becomes its characteristic stirrup shape during the 10th week, after which time the stapedial artery regresses. By the sixth month, the ossicles have achieved adult size; the middle ear cavity, the oval and round windows, and the tympanic membrane reach adult size at the time of birth.

Development of middle ear space and mastoid space

The tympanic cavity is covered by the tegmen tympani, which is an extension laterally of the otic capsule and medially from a band of fibrous tissue. The anterior epitympanic wall and the lateral tympanic cavity are formed from the tympanic process of the squamous temporal bone [4].

By 3 months of gestation, the mesenchyme filling the tympanic cavity becomes loose and vacuolated, allowing the tympanic cavity to expand. This expansion is complete by week 30; expansion of the epitympanum follows in the subsequent 4 weeks. The antrum extends laterally from the epitympanum beginning at 21 to 22 weeks, with near complete development by 34 weeks. Pneumatization of the mastoid air cells begins at approximately 33 weeks. Complete mastoid bone development occurs after birth. The lining epithelium expands the air cells, resulting in expansion of the antrum and the tympanic plate. The mastoid tip is not developed at birth but develops subsequently from the inferiorly directed traction of the sternocleidomastoid muscle, usually being complete by 1 year of age.

Inner ear development

The inner ear, consisting of the membranous labyrinth surrounded by a bony labyrinth, is adult size at the time of birth (except for changes in the periosteal layer and continued growth of the endolymphatic system). The membranous labyrinth (utricle, saccule, semicircular ducts, endolymphatic sac and duct, and cochlear duct), which is filled with endolymph, resides within the bony labyrinth, which is filled with perilymph. At 22 days of development, surface ectoderm on each side of the rhombencephalon thickens to form the otic placodes, which subsequently invaginate and form otocysts (otic and auditory vesicles), separating from the overlying ectoderm. Each vesicle divides into a ventral component that gives rise to the saccule and cochlear duct and a dorsal component that forms the utricle, semicircular canals, and endolymphatic duct. These epithelial structures are known as the membranous labyrinth [1–3,5].

In the sixth week of development, the cochlear duct forms from a tubular outgrowth of the saccule and penetrates surrounding mesenchyme to complete 2.5 turns by 8 weeks (Fig. 2). The ductus reuniens is the remaining stalk that connects the saccule and the newly formed cochlear duct. The mesenchyme surrounding the cochlear duct differentiates into cartilage, and in the 10th week, this cartilaginous shell undergoes vacuolization to create the scala vestibuli and scala tympani, both perilymph spaces. The epithelial cells of the cochlear duct differentiate into an inner ridge (eventual spiral limbus) and outer ridge (eventual organ of Corti). The cells in these two ridges secrete a gelatinous substance that becomes the tectorial membrane [4]. The cochlear modiolus, carrying the cochlear nerve, develops from membranous bone (Fig. 3). Bone deposition occurs within the modiolus between 20 and 21 weeks between the basal and second turns of the cochlea, and by week 25, ossification is nearly complete [6].

The semicircular canals begin as evaginations of the utricular part of the otic vesicle during the sixth week. The walls of these outpocketings come into contact with one another to create three semicircular canals. During week 7, the crista ampullaris, a ridge-like structure composed of neuroepithelial cells, forms at the dilated (ampullated) end of each canal. These ampullated ends open into the utricle. The neuroepithelium and cristae are complete by week 11 [1].

The utricle (an otolithic organ) develops from the dorsal pouch of the auditory vesicle, whereas the saccule (the other otolithic organ) is derived from the ventral pouch. They begin to develop at about week 6 and are complete by about week 8. Neuroepithelial cells, present in the macula of the utricle and saccule, contain type I and type II hair cells, like the cristae in the semicircular canals. Similar to the cristae, development of this neuroepithelium is complete by week 11 [1].

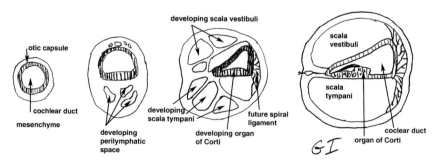

Fig. 2. Cochlear development. (*Adapted by* Glenn Isaacson, MD, from Moore KL, Persaud TVN. The developing human: clinically oriented embryology, 7th ed. Philadelphia: WB Saunders; 2003; with permission.)

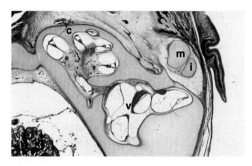

Fig. 3. Photomicrograph of axial section through fetal middle and inner ear at 11 weeks' gestation. c, cochlea; i, incus; m, malleus; v, vestibule. (*Courtesy of* Glenn Isaacson, MD, Philadelphia, PA.)

The eighth nerve ganglion is formed from cells from the otic vesicle during the fourth week of gestation. The eighth nerve ganglion then divides into the pars superior (which gives rise to the superior branch of the vestibular nerve) and the pars inferior (which becomes the inferior portion of the vestibular nerve and the cochlear nerve). These cells remain bipolar throughout life, with one process terminating in the brain stem and the peripheral part terminating in the sensory areas of the inner ear [1].

Anomalies of the middle ear

Congenital atresia of the external auditory canal and the spectrum of microtia and anotia are discussed elsewhere in this issue. In severe cases of external auditory canal atresia, a bony plate replaces the tympanic ring and forms the lateral wall of the middle ear cavity. It is important to recognize that external auditory canal atresia can be associated not only with pinna abnormalities but also with middle ear abnormalities. Because the external and middle ear share a common embryologic derivative—the first and second branchial arch—external ear abnormalities are often associated with middle ear abnormalities. A classification and scoring system to evaluate the severity of the middle ear abnormalities has been developed by Jahrsdoerfer [7] but is beyond the scope of this article. This scoring system is ideally used to assess surgical candidacy and potentially predict postoperative success.

Ossicular abnormalities are numerous and include absent or maldevelopment of any of the ossicles, with subsequent altered anatomy of other middle ear structures (such as the course of the facial nerve). Malleus head fixation, possibly the most common ossicular abnormality, occurs secondary to incomplete pneumatization of the epitympanum.

Congenital absence of the long process of the incus, which results in a near maximal conductive hearing loss, has been reported. The mode of transmission in a pedigree of three female patients was autosomal dominant mutation or X-linked dominant inheritance [8]. The authors' institution reported a rare case of isolated, congenital, bilateral absence of the incus in a 3-year-old [9]. In the reported cases, the use of middle ear prosthesis to reconstruct the ossicular chain has been successful in improving the hearing.

Congenital stapes disorders are often related to aberrant facial nerve development. During the crucial time period of 6 weeks post fertilization, if the facial nerve is displaced anteriorly, then the stapes are prevented from coming in contact with the otic capsule, resulting in a malformed stapes. Isolated congenital stapes ankylosis is a rare but reported entity that must be considered in a child who has a stable conductive hearing loss without other associated middle ear pathology [10]. An association of stapes fixation with perilymphatic gusher and profound or mixed hearing loss has been identified as an X-linked inheritance pattern within gene POU3F4 [11].

Isolated atresia of the oval window has been reported and can best be identified by high-resolution CT imaging in patients who have congenital conductive hearing loss [12,13]. A temporal bone study of nine patients noted oval window atresia to be associated with an aberrant course of the facial nerve, a malformed incus, and displaced stapes [13]. These patients had audiograms consistent with a conductive, sensorineural, or mixed hearing loss pattern; the role of imaging in establishing the diagnosis was essential [12,13]. Imaging with high-resolution CT should be strongly considered when a diagnosis of congenital conductive hearing loss is suspected [14,15].

Persistent stapedial artery has an interesting embryologic background. At approximately 10 weeks' gestation, the stapedial artery—a remnant of the second branchial arch—regresses, leaving the normally stirrup-shaped stapes. When this regression does not occur, the persistent artery travels above the stapes footplate, between the anterior and posterior stapes crura, to the fallopian canal toward the geniculate ganglion and dura. During a middle ear exploration for presumed otosclerosis or potential cochlear implantation, the surgeon must be aware of this potential embryologic maldevelopment. The course of the carotid artery may be altered when a persistent stapedial artery is identified; the carotid may be tethered by the stapedial artery and it may be more lateral and posterior than normal. Physical examination in patients with a persistent stapedial artery may show a pulsatile mass in the mesotympanum [16]. CT imaging findings of persistent stapedial artery include absence of the foramen spinosum on the ipsilateral side and abnormal soft tissue in the region of the tympanic segment of the facial nerve [16]. In one series, three of five cases of persistent stapedial artery were associated with an aberrant course of the internal carotid artery [16].

In addition to ossicular abnormalities, congenital cholesteatoma is attributed to alteration in normal embryologic development. The finding of a cholesteatoma in the anterior mesotympanum is controversial, although most investigators believe it is due to the epithelial rest theory in which there is failure of atrophy of epidermoid rests [17]. Epidermoid formation occurs during 10 to 33 weeks' gestation and subsequently involutes. The epidermoids persist as collections of stratified squamous epithelium in the anterior-superior portion of the middle ear and tympanic membrane and, when they produce keratin, congenital cholesteatoma develops [18].

A high-riding jugular bulb may be seen in asymptomatic patients or in patients who have a conductive hearing loss. It presents as a bluish hue behind an intact tympanic membrane and may be mistaken for a middle ear effusion. Patients may also complain of a venous hum or debilitating tinnitus. Selective ligation of the jugular vein has been noted to result in cessation of tinnitus in some patients [19]. CT scan can differentiate between middle ear effusion and a high-riding jugular bulb.

Congenital perilymphatic fistula has been associated with Mondini's deformity of the cochlea [3]. Sites of fistula include the oval window, fundus of the modiolus, fissulae ante fenstram, and round window [3]. Patients who have congenital perilymphatic fistula are at increased risk for bacterial meningitis [20]. Symptoms include fluctuating or progressive sensorineural or mixed hearing loss and intermittent unsteadiness or vertigo.

Middle ear exploration for anomalies of the middle ear

A study of the findings of middle ear explorations in 67 patients from the Hospital for Sick Children revealed 19 cases of stapes fixation and 42 patients who had ossicular malformation without stapes fixation [21]. Almost one half of operative patients showed no improvement in the air-bone gaps postoperatively [21]. Two thirds of patients who had a mobile stapes had a postoperative air-bone gap less than 30 dB.

An interesting association of middle and inner ear abnormalities in infants who had congenital heart defects was noted by Ulualp and colleagues [22]. Their study examined the histopathology of temporal bones in infants who had syndromic and nonsyndromic congenital cardiac defects and noted that middle and inner ear anomalies included malformed stapes, persistent stapedial artery, dehiscent facial nerve canal, and outer hair cell loss.

Anomalies of the inner ear

Inner ear anomalies are frequently found in patients who have sensorineural hearing loss (SNHL). These anomalies can be classified as involving the membranous portion of the labyrinth only or the bony and the membranous components. Again, the membranous labyrinth consists of the cochlear duct, semicircular ducts, utricle, saccule, and endolymphatic duct and sac. The bony labyrinth envelops the membranous labyrinth and consists of the cochlea, three semicircular canals, and the vestibule. Most inner ear anomalies accounting for SNHL are purely membranous; however, current imaging capabilities limit our ability to diagnose patients who have labyrinthine anomalies to those who have associated bony malformations, and purely membranous malformations can only be seen on histologic section.

Ever-improving imaging, however, including CT and MRI of the temporal bone, may show osseous anatomic abnormalities in up to 40% of patients who have SNHL [23].

As the ability to evaluate patients who have SNHL has improved, the classification of inner ear anomalies has changed. In 1791, using histopathologic findings, Mondini [24] described malformations of the cochlea in a deaf patient. His work was continued by others, including Alexander (1904) and Schuknecht [25]. Mondini described a specific cochlear malformation of incomplete partition, dilated vestibule, and large vestibular aqueduct (LVA) (Fig. 4) [26]. Several subsequent classification systems have described Mondini malformations as any osseous anomaly of the cochlea [27]. With the development of cochlear implantation, evaluation of patients as implant candidates has highlighted the need to distinguish between degrees of malformation of the cochlea. Also, the development of CT and MRI temporal bone imaging allows bony inner ear anomalies to be more easily identified. As a result, the classification of Mondini's malformation is now limited to the anomaly of the incomplete partition as it was originally described. The remaining cochlear malformations have been further classified.

Currently, the most common classification system of labyrinthine malformations is that which was introduced by Jackler and colleagues in 1987 [28]. This system proposed classification of inner ear anomalies based on their likely occurrence in embryogenesis. Based on radiographic and histologic studies, the most significant events in embryologic development of the labyrinth were noted to occur between the fourth and eighth weeks of gestation, with further maturation occurring up until birth and possibly beyond. Most inner ear malformations resemble histologic sections of the inner ear taken at different points in development, leading Jackler and

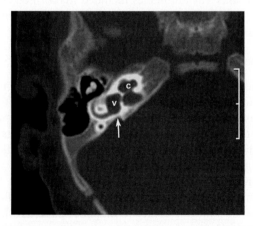

Fig. 4. Axial CT of Mondini malformation. Arrow indicates LVA. c, foreshortened cochlea; v, dilated vestibule.

colleagues [28] to conclude that malformations arise as a result of arrest in development at a specific point in embryogenesis.

Based on this system, malformations are divided into membranous alone or membranous and osseous anomalies. These malformations are further divided based on stage of embryologic arrest. Although their development occurs during the same time period, the development of the semicircular canals and cochlea are dependent on many genes, several of which are specific for the cochlea or the vestibular apparatus. Therefore, isolated arrest in the development of each of these structures can occur.

Although Jackler and colleagues' [28] classification system cannot account for the entire constellation of inner ear anomalies, it provides the most logical system of evaluating inner ear anomalies and communicating findings regarding these anomalies. Further divisions of cochlear anomalies have been proposed as imaging techniques have improved and genetic markers specific to the cochlear and vestibular systems have been discovered, and further classification can be expected as our ability to radiographically and clinically detect membranous anomalies improves.

Michel aplasia (complete labyrinthine aplasia)

The arrest of inner ear development before the fourth week of gestation results in complete aplasia of all inner ear structures. This rare anomaly was described by Michel in 1863 [25]. CT imaging shows an absence of inner ear structures. Rarely, complete aplasia can be confused with labyrinthitis ossificans. In this condition, the labyrinth is fully formed but obliterated. The lack of a promontory bulge in the middle ear on CT is seen in complete aplasia, whereas the promontory, although obliterated, is present in labyrinthitis ossificans. Less severe forms of labyrinthitis ossificans can also be detected with MRI. A recent study demonstrated that MRI is more sensitive in the detection of neo-ossification of the cochlear duct compared with high-resolution CT [29]. This distinction between cochlear aplasia and labyrinthitis obliterans becomes important when considering a patient for cochlear implantation because aplasia is an absolute contraindication, whereas implantation has been successful in some patients who have labyrinthitis ossificans [29].

Clinically, Michel aplasia has been associated with thalidomide exposure, anencephaly, and Klippel-Feil syndrome [5]. As expected, patients who have Michel anomaly present with profound SNHL. Although these patients are not candidates for cochlear implantation, they may be candidates for brain stem implantation in the future [30].

Cochlear anomalies

Common cavity deformity

Failure of the cochlear and vestibular apparatus to develop early in the fourth week of gestation results in a common cavity deformity. In this anomaly, the membranous labyrinth is poorly differentiated and situated in a large common cavity (Fig. 5) [31]. The labyrinthine segment of the facial nerve can be displaced anteromedially. On axial CT, a common cavity can be differentiated from lateral semicircular canal dysplasia by its anterior position with respect to the internal auditory canal [5].

Hearing loss in patients who have a common cavity is generally in the severe to profound range. Although cochlear implantation has been successfully performed on these patients, results vary depending on degree of membranous and neural development. Surgically, cerebrospinal fluid or perilymphatic leaks are common and need to be addressed with the patient preoperatively [32].

Cochlear aplasia

Failure in labyrinth development in the fifth week of gestation results in cochlear aplasia. This is a rare anomaly whereby the cochlea fails to develop in the presence of vestibular development. Although present, the vestibule and semicircular canals are abnormal and distinguished from the cochlea by their position posterior to the internal auditory canal. These patients present with profound SNHL, and implantation may be precluded by lack of an auditory nerve [33].

Cochlear hypoplasia

Arrest of development in the sixth week of gestation results in cochlear hypoplasia. On CT imaging, the cochlea may appear round and undeveloped, usually measuring 6 mm in height compared with a normal cochlea of 10 to 12 mm. In severe cases, the labyrinthine segment of the facial nerve can be displaced anteromedially [31]. These patients present with differing degrees of hearing loss depending on the exact time of arrest within the sixth week. Patients who have greater differentiation of the membranous labyrinth and more neuroepithelial elements have greater hearing. Hearing

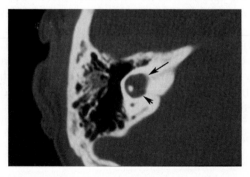

Fig. 5. Axial CT of common cavity defect (*arrow* and *arrowhead*). (*Courtesy of* Glenn Isaacson, MD, Philadelphia, PA.)

results following cochlear implantation also depend on the degree of membranous differentiation.

Mondini malformation (incomplete partition)

Incomplete partition of the cochlea is the most common cochlear malformation seen on imaging, accounting for up to one half of all bony cochlear anomalies [5]. It is frequently associated with the presence of an enlarged vestibular aqueduct (EVA). The spectrum of malformations classified as incomplete partition malformation ranges from a cystic cochlea lacking all interscalar septae and modiolus to a cochlea with a normal basal turn but lacking a complete 2.5 turns. The first entity has been referred to as pseudo-Mondini malformation or cystic cochleovestibular malformation. The second is the classically described Mondini malformation. Several investigators have proposed classifying these two entities separately because the degree of hearing loss in true Mondini malformation is typically less severe than in the cystic cochleovestibular malformation [27,34].

As originally described, Mondini malformation consists of an incomplete partition of the cochlea. Instead of its usual 2.5 turns, the cochlea has 1.5 turns, with an absent interscalar septum between the middle and apical turn. Embryologically, this absence corresponds to arrest in development during the seventh week of gestation. Pseudo-Mondini malformation have occurs earlier in the seventh week than the more developed Mondini malformation.

Stapes footplate anomalies and modiolar defects have also been found in association with Mondini malformation, predisposing these patients to the risk of perilymphatic fistula and meningitis. Hearing loss depends on the degree of development of the membranous labyrinth. Seventh nerve anomalies are typically found when stapes anomalies are present, with displacement of the second genu anteriorly and inferiorly [32]. Mondini malformations have been associated with several syndromes including Waardenburg, DiGeorge, and Pendred. Pendrin gene defects have also been seen in nonsyndromic SNHL cases associated with EVA [35].

Large vestibular aqueduct

LVA, also known as EVA, is the most common inner ear anomaly seen on temporal bone imaging in patients who have SNHL. Although it is agreed to be the most common radiographic finding, the definition of LVA varies. It is most commonly described as an aqueduct that measures 1.5 mm or greater at the midpoint between its internal and external aperture; however, other investigators define it as an aqueduct having a diameter greater than 2 mm, with the measurement taken at its widest point or at the external aperture [36,37]. A large endolymphatic sac, with or without the presence of LVA, is also associated with hearing loss. Although LVA can be detected with CT (Fig. 6) and MRI, the entire endolymphatic sac can be seen only with MRI [29].

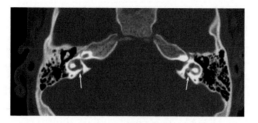

Fig. 6. Axial CT of EVAs (*arrows*).

LVA is found in association with cochlear anomalies, most commonly in-complete partition. Cases of LVA in isolation have been reported; however, this is disputed [38]. One argument in favor of the isolated LVA is based on the embryogenesis of the vestibular aqueduct. A histologic study by Pyle [36] demonstrated progressive growth of the aqueduct throughout gestation, whereas growth of the remaining labyrinth was virtually complete by the second trimester. Therefore, an isolated LVA could occur following normal development of the cochlea and semicircular canals. Opposing arguments, however, have been raised, proposing developmental arrest at 5 weeks as the etiology of LVA [32].

LVA is often associated with Pendred syndrome. Pendred syndrome, characterized by euthyroid goiter and SNHL, is the most common syn-drome with associated SNHL, accounting for 10% of patients who have syndromic hearing loss. Mutations in the Pendrin gene (PDS, SLC26A4) cause Pendred syndrome but are also responsible for a nonsyndromic form of recessive SNHL (DFNB4). In the nonsyndromic form, the patients have temporal bone anomalies without associated thyroid goiter or detectable abnormalities of thyroid function. The findings of LVA can also be found in X-linked mixed deafness with gusher (DFN3, POU3F4) and branchio-oto-renal syndrome (associated with mutations in the EYA1 and SIX1 genes) [39]. In each syndrome, associated cochlear malformations are common.

The clinical presentation of the hearing loss in patients who have EVA is variable. The hearing loss may be sensorineural or mixed. Frequently, pa-tients have normal hearing at birth and experience progressive or fluctuating hearing loss. Sudden hearing loss is also seen spontaneously or with even mild head trauma. Forty percent of patients who have LVA develop pro-found SNHL [5]. Proposed mechanisms for hearing loss include membrane rupture causing a change in electrolyte homeostasis versus increased pres-sure forcing cerebrospinal fluid through the cochlear duct [37,40].

Hearing preservation procedures in patients who have EVA have been at-tempted through endolymphatic sac shunts, occlusion, or decompression; however, the results were disappointing, with 50% to 100% of the patients developing worse hearing loss following the procedure [1,41]. As a result, surgical intervention is not recommended. Currently, patients are advised to avoid activities that have high risk for head trauma or pressure changes, such as flying or diving, although the incidence of a permanent change in the hearing from these activities remains unclear.

Vestibular anomalies

The most common abnormality of the vestibular apparatus is aplasia or dysplasia of the lateral semicircular canal. Lateral semicircular canal dysplasia is reported by some investigators to be the second most common osseous inner ear anomaly after LVA [24,42]. The lateral semicircular canal is more often involved due to its later embryonic development than the superior and posterior canals. Vestibular malformations frequently present in association with cochlear malformations and LVAs because their development occurs during the same weeks of gestation.

Patients who have lateral semicircular canal dysplasia may present with sensorineural, mixed, or conductive hearing loss. It occurs in isolation or is associated with a syndrome. A commonly associated syndrome is CHARGE syndrome. CHARGE syndrome has a characteristic inner ear finding exhibiting semicircular canal aplasia in association with a stenotic cochlear aperture, underdeveloped vestibule, and incomplete partition of the cochlea.

Membranous anomalies

Membranous labyrinthine anomalies occur in isolation and in combination with all bony labyrinthine anomalies. They account for a large percentage of patients who have SNHL but, because of limitations in imaging, can only be inferred without histologic sectioning. As previously mentioned, the membranous labyrinth is divided into two components: the pars superior and the pars inferior. The pars superior forms the semicircular canals, endolymphatic duct, and utricle; the pars inferior becomes the saccule and cochlear duct. Anomalies can involve an isolated portion of the membranous labyrinth, one division, or the entire labyrinth.

Bing-Siebenmann malformation (cochleosaccular dysplasia)

The Bing-Siebenmann malformation is an isolated membranous malformation characterized by membranous labyrinthine aplasia or dysplasia with a well-formed bony capsule. On histopathologic section, the cochlear duct has a poorly developed organ of Corti with an abnormal stria vascularis, and collapse of Reissner's membrane. The saccule and macula are also poorly developed. Clinically, patients who have Bing-Siebenmann malformation have profound SNHL. This malformation has been seen in patients diagnosed with Usher syndrome and Jervell and Lange-Nielsen syndrome.

Scheibe malformation

Scheibe malformation is the most common membranous inner ear malformation. It results from a defect in the development of the pars inferior, resulting in a malformed organ of Corti and saccule. Histologically, there is a partial or complete aplasia of the organ of Corti and collapse of the cochlear duct. Clinically, the Scheibe malformation presents with severe to profound SNHL. It is most often associated with Usher syndrome but is also seen with Jervell and Lange-Nielsen, Refsum disease, Waardenburg syndrome, and trisomy 18. Inheritance in an autosomal recessive fashion with a gene defect on chromosome 1q32 has also been demonstrated [5].

Alexander malformation

The least severe membranous malformation was described by Alexander in 1904. It involves an otherwise normal labyrinth with the exception of a dysplastic basal turn of the cochlea. The Alexander malformation is found in association with hereditary high-frequency SNHL.

Summary

Understanding the anatomy and embryologic basis of middle and inner ear malformations is an important aspect of the diagnosis and treatment of patients who have congenital hearing loss. Knowledge of embryology helps to predict anomalies of the ossicles, labyrinth, and facial nerve and aids in planning of medical or surgical intervention. This understanding continues to evolve as imaging techniques, genetic testing, and treatment options improve.

References

[1] Kenna MA, Hirose K. Embryology and developmental anatomy of the ear. In: Bluestone CD, Stool SE, Alper CM, et al, editors. Pediatric otolaryngology. 4th edition. Philadelphia: Saunders; 2003. p. 129–45 [Chapter 8].
[2] Sadler TW. Langman's medical embryology. 7th edition. Baltimore (MD): Williams & Wilkins; 1995.
[3] Wareing MJ, Lalwani AK, Jackler RK. Development of the ear. In: Bailey B, Johnson JT, Newlands SD, et al, editors. Head and Neck Surgery-Otolaryngology. 4th edition. Philadelphia: Lippincott Williams and Wilkins; 2006. Chapter 128.
[4] Pearson AA. Developmental anatomy of the ear. In: English GM, editor. Otolaryngology. Revised edition. New York: Harper Medical; 1988. p. 1–68.
[5] Reilly GP, Lalwani AK, Jackler RK. Congenital anomalies of the inner ear. In: Lalwani AK, Grundfast KM, editors. Pediatric otology and neurotology. Philadelphia: Lippincott-Raven; 1998. p. 201–10.
[6] Gulya AJ. Developmental anatomy of the temporal bone and skull base. In: Glasscock ME, Gulya AJ, editors. Surgery of the ear. 5th edition. Hamilton (Ontario): BC Decker; 2002. p. 3–33 [Chapter 1].

[7] Jahrsdoerfer RA, Yeakley JW, Aguilar EA, et al. Grading system for the selection of patients with congenital aural atresia. Am J Otol 1992;13(1):6–12.

[8] Wehrs RE. Congenital absence of the long process of the incus. Laryngoscope 1999;109(2 Pt 1): 192–7.

[9] Rahbar R, Neault MW, Kenna MA. Congenital absence of the incus bilaterally without other otologic abnormalities: a new case report. Ear Nose Throat J 2002;81(4):274–6, 278.

[10] Nandapalan V, Tos M. Isolated congenital stapes ankylosis: an embryologic survey and literature review. Am J Otol 2000;21(1):71–80.

[11] de Kok YJM, van der Maarel SM, Bitner-Glindzicz M, et al. Association between X-linked mixed deafness and mutations in the POU domain gene POU3F4. Science 1995;267:685–8.

[12] Booth TN, Vezina LG, Karcher G, et al. Imaging and clinical evaluation of isolated atresia of the oval window. AJNR Am J Neuroradiol 2000;21(1):171–4.

[13] Zeifer B, Sabini P, Sonne J. Congenital absence of the oval window: radiologic diagnosis and associated anomalies. AJNR Am J Neuroradiol 2000;21(2):322–7.

[14] Tan TY, Goh JP. Imaging of congenital middle ear deafness. Ann Acad Med Singap 2003; 32(4):495–9.

[15] Watanabe A, Miyahsima H, Kobashi T, et al. CT findings of bilateral congenital absence of the long process of the incus. Neuroradiology 2004;46(10):859–61.

[16] Silbergleit R, Quint DJ, Mehta BA, et al. The persistent stapedial artery. AJNR Am J Neuroradiol 2000;21(3):572–7.

[17] Kazahaya K, Potsic WP. Congenital cholesteatoma. Curr Opin Otolaryngol Head Neck Surg 2004;12(5):398–403.

[18] Levenson MJ, Michaels L, Parisier SC, et al. Congenital cholesteatomas in children: an embryologic correlation. Laryngoscope 1988;98:949–55.

[19] Golueke PJ, Panetta T, Sclafani S, et al. Tinnitus originating from an abnormal jugular bulb: treatment by jugular vein ligation. J Vasc Surg 1987;6(3):248–51.

[20] Claros P, Guirado C, Claros A, et al. Association of spontaneous anterior fossa CSF rhinorrhea and congenital perilymphatic fistula in a patient with recurrent meningitis. Int J Pediatr Otorhinolaryngol 1993;27(1):65–71.

[21] Raveh E, Hu W, Papsin BC, et al. Congenital conductive hearing loss. J Laryngol Otol 2002; 116(2):92–6.

[22] Ulualp SO, Wright GC, Roland PS. Spectrum of middle and inner ear abnormalities in infants with congenital heart defects. Otolaryngol Head Neck Surg 2005;133(2):260–8.

[23] Purcell D, Johnson J, Fischbein N, et al. Establishment of normative cochlear and vestibular measurements to aid in the diagnosis of inner ear malformations. Otolaryngol Head Neck Surg 2003;128:78–87.

[24] Mondini C. Anatomia surdi nedi section. De Bononiensi Scientarum et Artum Institutio Atque Academea Commentarii Bologna 1791;7:28, 419.

[25] Schuknecht HF. Developmental defects. In: Pathology of the ear. 2nd edition. Philadelphia: Lea and Febiger; 1993. p. 115–89 [Chapter 4].

[26] Wu CC, Chen YS, Chen PJ, et al. Common clinical features of children with enlarged vestibular aqueduct and Mondini dysplasia. Laryngoscope 2005;115:132–7.

[27] Sennaroglu L, Saatci I. A new classification of cochleovestibular malformations. Laryngoscope 2002;112:2230–41.

[28] Jackler RK, Luxford WM, House WF. Congenital malformations of the inner ear: a classification based on organogenesis. Laryngoscope 1987;97(Suppl 40):2–14.

[29] Parry DA, Booth T, Roland PS. Advantages of magnetic resonance imaging over computed tomography in preoperative evaluation of pediatric cochlear implant candidates. Otol Neurotol 2005;26:976–82.

[30] Colletti V, Carner M, Fiorino F, et al. Hearing restoration with auditory brainstem implant in three children with cochlear nerve aplasia. Otol Neurotol 2002;23(5):682–93.

[31] Romo LV, Curtin HD. Anomalous facial nerve canal with cochlear malformation. Am J Neuroradiol 2001;2:838–44.

[32] Papsin BC. Cochlear implantation in children with anomalous cochleovestibular anatomy. Laryngoscope 2005;115(Suppl):1–25.

[33] Mylanus EAM, Rotteveel LJ, Leeuw RL. Congenital malformation of the inner ear and pediatric cochlear implantation. Otol Neurotol 2004;25:308–17.

[34] Phelps PD. Mondini and pseudo-Mondini. Clin Otolaryngol 1990;15:99–101.

[35] Albert S, Blons H, Jonard L, et al. SLC26A4 gene is frequently involved in nonsyndromic hearing impairment with enlarged vestibular aqueduct in Caucasian populations. Eur J Hum Genet 2006;14(6):773–9.

[36] Pyle GM. Embryological development and large vestibular aqueduct syndrome. Laryngoscope 2000;110:1837–42.

[37] Arjmand EM, Webber A. Audiometric findings in children with a large vestibular aqueduct. Arch Otolaryngol Head Neck Surg 2004;130:1169–74.

[38] Lemmerling MM, Mancuso AA, Antonelli PJ, et al. Normal modiolus: CT appearance in patients with a large vestibular aqueduct. Radiology 1997;204:213–9.

[39] Van Camp G, Smith RJH. Hereditary hearing loss homepage. Available at: http://webhost.ua.ac.be/hhh/. Accessed September 26, 2006.

[40] Lai CC, Shiao AS. Chronological changes of hearing in pediatric patients with large vestibular aqueduct syndrome. Laryngoscope 2004;114:832–8.

[41] Park AH, Kou B, Hotaling A, et al. Clinical course of pediatric congenital inner ear malformations. Laryngoscope 2000;110:1715–8.

[42] Johnson J, Lalwani AK. Sensorineural and conductive hearing loss associated with lateral semicircular canal malformation. Laryngoscope 2000;110:1673–9.

ELSEVIER
SAUNDERS

Otolaryngol Clin N Am
40 (2007) 97–112

OTOLARYNGOLOGIC
CLINICS
OF NORTH AMERICA

Congenital Nasal Malformations

Wasyl Szeremeta, MD*, Tejas Dinesh Parikh, BS,
Jeffrey S. Widelitz, MD

Temple University School of Medicine, Philadelphia, PA, USA

Nasal embryology

External nose formation begins when the embryonic stomodeum appears during the fourth and fifth weeks of gestation, delineating the center of the face. The stomodeum is surrounded by the maxillary, mandibular, and frontal prominences [1]. On the lateral aspects of the frontal prominence, neural crest cells proliferate and form the nasal placodes. The nasal placodes invaginate to form the olfactory pit, which further invaginates to form the nasal processes (Fig. 1).

Forming on the outer edge of the pits are the lateral nasal processes. Those on the inner side are the medial nasal processes [2]. The lateral rounded angles of the medial prominences are the globular processes. The globular processes continue (Figs. 2–4) posteriorly as plates termed the *nasal laminae*. The nasal laminae fuse with the nasofrontal process in an anterior to posterior direction, creating the nasal septum and initially partitioning the nasal cavity into left and right divisions [3,4]. The nasal septum continues to grow posteriorly and begins fusion with the palatine processes during the ninth week of gestation. Chondrification and ossification begin around the twelfth week, but ossification does not fully complete until puberty [2].

The globular processes of the medial prominences then fuse with the maxillary processes, forming the philtrum and the columella. The maxillary processes also give rise to the lower portion of the lateral walls of the nasal cavity and the posterior borders of the nares. The nares are initially filled with epithelium, which eventually breaks down by the 24th week, leading to the permanent openings (Fig. 5) [1].

Ectoderm of the nasal sac contacts ectoderm of the roof of the mouth, forming the oronasal septum. Attenuation of this septum leads to creation

* Corresponding author.
E-mail address: wasyl@ent.temple.edu (W. Szeremeta).

0030-6665/07/$ - see front matter © 2007 Elsevier Inc. All rights reserved.
doi:10.1016/j.otc.2006.10.008

4.5 Week Embryo

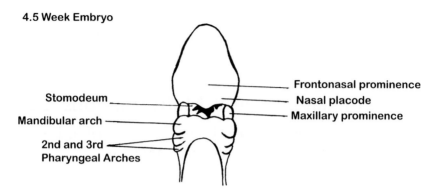

Fig. 1. Embryo at 4.5 weeks. Nasal placodes are found on both sides of the frontonasal prominence. (*Courtesy of* Tatiana Skvirski, after Sadler TW. Langman's medical embryology. 8th edition. Philadelphia: Lippincott Williams & Wilkins; 2000.)

of the oronasal membrane separating the nasal cavity from the pharynx. The oronasal membrane then undergoes degeneration, forming the choanae. Beginning at 6.5 weeks, lateral nasal wall development occurs. The inferior concha appears above the palatine processes. As the nasal cavity heightens, ectodermal folds appear in the ethmoid region and give rise to superior, middle, and inferior conchae (Fig. 6) [1].

Nasal cleft deformities

Nasal cleft deformities include nasal clefting, cleft lip, and cleft palate. Cleft lip and palate are addressed elsewhere in this issue. This section discusses nasal cleft defects, associated esthetic and airflow complications, and the repair of these malformations.

5 week embryo

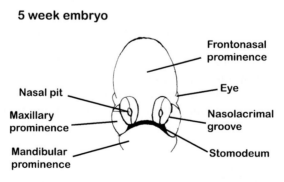

Fig. 2. Embryo at 5 weeks. (*Courtesy of* Tatiana Skvirski, after Sadler TW. Langman's medical embryology. 8th edition. Philadelphia: Lippincott Williams & Wilkins; 2000.)

6 week embryo

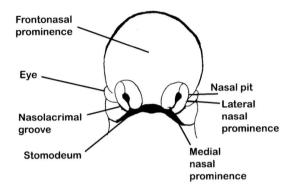

Fig. 3. Embryo at 6 weeks. (*Courtesy of* Tatiana Skvirski, after Sadler TW. Langman's medical embryology. 8th edition. Philadelphia: Lippincott Williams & Wilkins; 2000.)

Nasal defects associated with cleft lip and palate

Nasal deformities are commonly seen in children who have cleft lip. In general, the worse the cleft lip, the worse the nasal deformity [2]. According to facial development theories, cleft palate begins to occur at 35 days' gestation, leading to nasal septal deviation. The nasal defects can be unilateral or bilateral. In unilateral cleft, the premaxilla and maxilla tethers the septum, causing it to deviate. As embryogenesis continues, maxillary growth

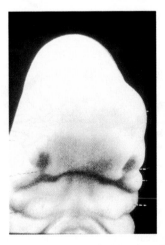

Fig. 4. Scanning electron micrograph of the craniofacial region of a human embryo at Carnegie stage 16—about 37 days. (*From* Moore KL, Persaud TVN, Shiota K. Color atlas of clinical embryology. 2nd edition. Philadelphia (PA): WB Saunders; 1994. p. 132; with permission.)

7 week embryo   **10 week embryo**

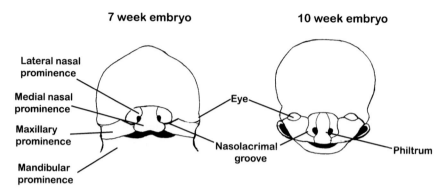

Fig. 5. Embryo at 7 weeks (*left*) and at 10 weeks (*right*). (*Courtesy of* Tatiana Skvirski, after Sadler TW. Langman's medical embryology. 8th edition. Philadelphia: Lippincott Williams & Wilkins; 2000.)

is also hindered by the tethered septum, leading to maxillary hypoplasia in the caudal-cranial and anterior-posterior directions [5,6].

When a cleft lip is unilateral, the medial nasal crus is medially and inferiorly rotated. Due to the maxillary bone hypoplasia, the nasal ala is retrodisplaced and the nostril is flat and flared. The nasal tip may appear uneven,

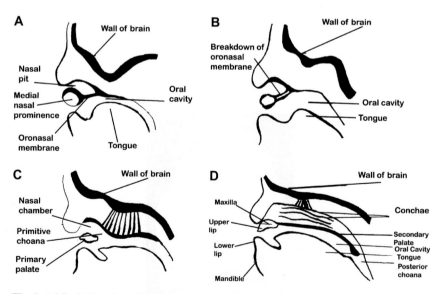

Fig. 6. (*A*) Sagittal section of 6-week embryo through lower rim of the medial nasal prominence and nasal pit. (*B*) Sagittal section of 6-week embryo through lower rim of the medial nasal prominence and nasal pit with oronasal membrane beginning to resorb. (*C*) Sagittal section of 7-week embryo with primitive nasal cavity communicating with the oral cavity. (*D*) Sagittal section of 9-week embryo showing separate oral and nasal cavities. (*Courtesy of* Tatiana Skvirski, after Sadler TW. Langman's medical embryology. 8th edition. Philadelphia: Lippincott Williams & Wilkins; 2000.)

wide, or boxy. The bases of the nares are widened, and the caudal septum and nasal spine are deviated to the nonaffected part of the nose. When a bilateral cleft defect is present, all the previously mentioned defects are present, along with a shortened columella and a relative prognathism due the bilaterally hypoplastic maxilla [2]. In some patients, the floor of the nasal cavity is absent [7].

Controversy surrounds the most appropriate timing of correction of cleft lip and nose deformities. At times, it may be beneficial to delay correction until facial growth is complete and nasal structures have fully matured. When the deformity is causing inadequate airflow and respiratory distress, however, the defect should be repaired earlier [2,6,7]. Because neonates are preferential nose breathers, early repair is often indicated [8,9].

Piriform aperture stenosis

Piriform aperture stenosis (PAS) is rare and subtle. Thus, it often overlooked as a cause of respiratory distress in neonates. PAS results from bony overgrowth of the nasal process of the maxilla, narrowing the anterior bony opening of the nose. This narrowing can cause increased nasal resistance and cyclic cyanotic periods [2,7]. The disorder usually presents in the initial few months of life. It may occur alone or in association with holoprosencephaly. A solitary maxillary central incisor may serve as a clue that additional significant abnormalities of the midface, orbits, and brain are present (Fig. 7) [7,10].

PAS is often found incidentally on intranasal examination. Axial CT is helpful in differentiating PAS from choanal atresia, demonstrating anterior bony nasal stenosis (Fig. 8) [7]. The differential diagnosis of anterior nasal obstruction includes nasal mucosa edema, obstruction of the nasal passage by a nasolacrimal duct cyst, or hypoplasia of the nasal alae [9].

Respiratory distress from PAS can be managed using an oral airway or a McGovern nipple, supplemented by humidified oxygen and nasal decongestants. Mild stenosis improves with growth and may never require

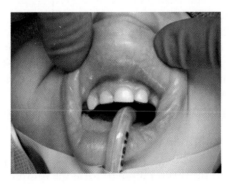

Fig. 7. Central maxillary incisor with PAS.

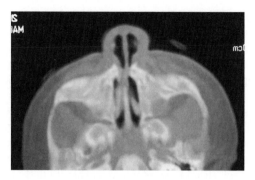

Fig. 8. CT of PAS.

surgery. When a neurologic deficit is suspected, MRI can help to rule out associated structural brain defects [11]. The neonate may be discharged from the hospital when an artificial airway is no longer needed and oral intake is adequate [7,10,11]. Respiratory status should be carefully monitored.

Surgery is indicated for persistent respiratory distress with cyanosis or apnea, or with poor feeding [10]. Repair is performed using a sublabial approach to the premaxilla. The narrowed nasal aperture is enlarged by submucosal drill-out of the nasal process of the maxilla. Care must be taken to preserve the nasolacrimal ducts and forming teeth [2]. Nasal stenting is usually employed for 1 to 6 weeks to prevent recurrent stenosis [10]. Extended postoperative follow-up is necessary to look for restenosis.

Nasal dermoid cysts

Midline congenital lesions of the nose are rare, affecting 1:20,000 to 1:40,000 newborns [12]. Nasal dermoid cysts are the most common of these congenital midline nasal defects and may present as noncompressible masses over the nasal dorsum with an associated midline pit. These cysts often present at birth or in early childhood. Masses and pits may appear anywhere from the glabella to the nasal columella. Sixty percent are located on the lower nasal dorsum. Thirty percent are intranasal and 10% are combined. Usually, nasal dermoids terminate in a single subcutaneous tract with hair at the opening. They may secrete sebaceous material or pus, if inflamed. They may cause recurrent septal abscesses or osteomyelitis or broaden the nasal root. With intracranial extension, infected nasal dermoids may lead to meningitis or brain abscess (Figs. 9 and 10) [13].

Grunwald [14] proposed a theory for midline nasal dermoid formation in 1910. At approximately 8 weeks of gestation, a dural diverticulum protrudes through the nasal and frontal bones to enter the space between the nasal bones and nasal capsule. As the nasal processes of the frontal bones grow, they surround the diverticulum to form the foramen cecum and therefore separate the dura from the skin. Normally, the diverticulum involutes,

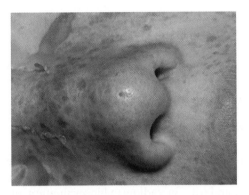

Fig. 9. External opening to nasal dermoid.

but incomplete closure of the path of the diverticulum results in a persistent attachment of the dura to the dermis. As the dura recedes, it pulls nasal ectoderm upward, which results in trapped epithelium along the diverticulum path. Proliferation of the trapped elements produces a dermoid containing glands and hair [15].

In addition to a dermoid cyst, the differential diagnosis of a midline nasal mass also includes gliomas and encephaloceles that are differentiated by clinical and imaging characteristics. A glioma is diagnosed whenever there is extracranial brain matter without the herniation of dura. An encephalocele herniates through a bony defect and consists of meninges and brain matter [13,15]. Encephaloceles sometimes transilluminate; nasal dermoids

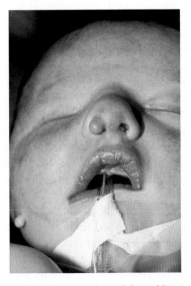

Fig. 10. Internal nasal dermoid.

do not. Encephaloceles enlarge with straining or crying (Furstenburg sign); lesions without an intracranial connection (dermoids or gliomas) lack this sign.

Although nasal dermoids are not associated with any named clinical syndromes, other congenital anomalies such as cleft defects, aural atresias, and hydrocephalus have been reported in up to 41% of cases of nasal dermoids [12]. The presence of other congenital anomalies increases the frequency of intracranial extension from 31% to 65% according to Wardinksi [16].

A thorough preoperative radiographic evaluation is necessary to look for intracranial extension and to guide surgical plans. CT and MRI have become the "gold standard" in radiographic evaluation of nasal dermoids. The findings on CT most consistent with intracranial involvement are an enlarged foramen cecum or bifid crista galli [13]. Some investigators, however, have found many preoperative false positives by these criteria [17]. High-resolution MRI should be obtained with T1, fat-suppression, T2, or fast-spin echo sequences. The use of contrast differentiates between avascular dermoids and enhancing lesions such as hemangiomas and vascular teratomas. It is important to note that the crista galli in infants is unossified and does not contain marrow fat. Any high-intensity signal on T1-weighted images in the vicinity of the crista galli in a newborn should suggest the possibility of an intracranial dermoid [18].

Nasal dermoids are treated surgically. Early treatment with complete excision of the lesion and tract prevents recurrence and avoids further distortion of the nose [15]. Failing to excise the complete tract may result in the recurrence of the dermoid or the formation of an abscess, osteomyelitis, or meningitis [15]. Denoyelle and colleagues [12] reported a recurrence rate of 5.5% (2/36 patients) for nasal dermoids in their series. Pollock [19] reviewed the surgical treatment of the nasal dermoid cyst and recommended four criteria for a surgical approach. First, the surgical approach should permit access to all midline cysts and readily permit medial and lateral osteotomies, if required. Second, the surgical exposure should favor the rapid repair of cribriform defects, should they be present, and would permit control of cerebrospinal fluid rhinorrhea, if it develops. Third, the surgical approach should allow reconstruction of the nasal dorsum, if it is required. Fourth, the approach should offer the probability of acceptable scar formation [13,15]. If frozen section analysis of the tract before it enters the skull base demonstrates fibrous tissue only, with no evidence of an epithelial tract, then the residual tract can be ligated without the need for formal excision through a transcranial approach [15].

Weiss and colleagues [20] described the use of endoscopic removal of nasal dermoids in two cases. They recommended the use of this technique when the dermoid is located within the nasal cavity and there is little or no cutaneous involvement. This technique can be combined with a small external midline excision of a cutaneous punctum [15].

Choanal atresia and stenosis

In 1755, Roederer first described a condition now known as congenital choanal atresia [21]. With a prevalence of 1 in 8000 births, choanal atresia is the most common major congenital anomaly of the nose. It is twice as common in girls as in boys [7].

The choanae are formed in the embryo by the degeneration of the bucconasal septum during the fifth or sixth week of gestation [21]. Choanal atresia results when the bucconasal membrane fails to degenerate. The four parts of the anatomic deformity include a narrow nasal cavity, lateral bony obstruction by the lateral pterygoid plate, medial obstruction caused by thickening of the vomer, and membranous obstruction [2]. Endoscopic views of a normal posterior choana and one with bilateral choanal atresia are depicted in Fig. 11.

Symptoms that should raise suspicion of bilateral choanal atresia include severe airway obstruction with cyclic cyanosis (cyanosis when the mouth is closed, resolving with crying or open-mouth posture). Suckling may be impossible in the neonate because the only airway (the mouth) is blocked [22].

Unilateral atresia is much harder to diagnose and may be overlooked for many years. Two thirds of choanal atresia cases are unilateral, with the right side being more commonly affected than the left. Choanal atresia is suspected at birth when a 5 or 6 French catheter cannot be passed through the nasal cavity into the nasopharynx. Qualitative measure of nasal airflow as the movement of a wisp of cotton under the nostrils or fogging of mirror add support to the clinical diagnosis. A colored solution placed in the anterior nares should pass into the pharynx in a short time when the choanae are patent [21]. The defect can be imaged using plain radiographs with contrast material in the nose, but the procedure of choice is CT with or without contrast (Fig. 12).

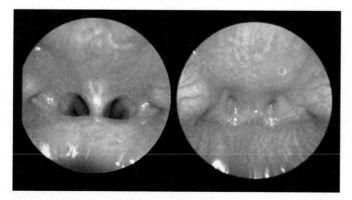

Fig. 11. The normal neonatal nasopharynx (*left*) and bilateral congenital posterior choanal atresia (*right*) in a newborn baby. (*From* Benjamin B. Diagnostic laryngology—adults and children. Philadelphia (PA): WB Saunders; 1989. p. 82; with permission.)

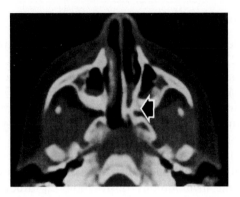

Fig. 12. Axial CT scan demonstrating a complete atresia of the left posterior choana. (*From* Benjamin B. Diagnostic laryngology—adults and children. Philadelphia (PA): WB Saunders; 1989. p. 83; with permission.)

CT confirms the clinical diagnosis and defines the extent of the defect [21]. Rigid or flexible endoscopy is useful when the nasal cavity is large enough for good visualization [2].

Half of infants who have unilateral choanal atresia and 60% of infants who have bilateral atresia present with other congenital anomalies. The most common of these anomalies is the CHARGE syndrome [21]. Malformations include:

Coloboma of the iris or choroid
Heart defect such as atrial septal defect or a conotruncal lesion
Atresia of the choanae
Retarded growth and development
Genitourinary abnormalities such as cryptorchidism, microphallus, or hydronephrosis
Ear defects with associated deafness

In children who present with the defects of CHARGE syndrome, 50% will have some form of choanal atresia. Patients who have choanal atresia should also be examined for the possible coexistence of Treacher Collins syndrome [2,22].

Treatment for bilateral choanal atresia is surgical. Initially, management requires airway support by positioning, by an oral airway, or by tracheotomy. A small feeding tube is often placed transorally for nutritional support [23].

Among the approaches to choanal atresia repair, transnasal puncture has fallen out of favor because of an unacceptable rate of recurrence. The transseptal technique creates a window in the nasal septum anterior to the atretic plate. The transpalatal approach provides excellent exposure and has a high success rate. Still, it requires it a lengthy procedure, may have significant blood loss, and can cause a palatal fistula [21].

Endoscopes have changed the approach to surgical correction of congenital choanal atresia in the past decade. Stankiewicz [24] reported the use of endoscopic instruments for choanal atresia repair. Three of four patients had good results in his series using an otologic drill and conventional instruments under endoscopic guidance. Endoscopic repair is now practiced following the development of pediatric-sized instruments originally designed for endoscopic sinus surgery. Power-suction soft tissue shavers and drills are believed to be less traumatic to nasal tissue and allow better healing. These powered instruments facilitate surgery by removing blood and debris during dissection, improving visualization and safety [25].

The transnasal endoscopic approach has combined the advantages of the traditional transnasal and transpalatal approaches without their disadvantages. The advantages include clear vision of operative field and accurate removal of the atretic plate and posterior vomerine bone without damage to surrounding structures. The procedure is applicable in all age groups, especially newborns, without interruption of maxillary growth centers [26].

Many investigators have advocated postoperative stenting for 4 to 6 weeks because this is the time necessary for the re-epithelization of the neochoana [27]. Some investigators have reported postoperative stenting to be unnecessary. Commercial stents are available or one can make a custom stent from a polyvinylchloride endotracheal tube. Mitomycin has been used in anecdotal cases to limit the narrowing of the surgically opened choanae secondary to scarring.

Regardless of which surgical technique is used, the goal is to create as large an opening as possible without injury to the structures found in the lateral wall of the choana. Even when an ample choanal opening is created, some patients require subsequent dilatations [13].

Congenital syndromes with malformed nasal structures

The presence of one craniofacial abnormality often indicates the existence of other anomalies that combine to characterize a disease or a syndrome. A common characteristic of many of the craniofacial abnormalities is maxillary hypoplasia. A small maxilla may produce a constricted nasal cavity, inadequate for respiration [7].

Crouzon syndrome

Crouzon syndrome was described in 1912. It is characterized by craniosynostosis, midface retrusion, and proptosis [28]. Crouzon syndrome is an autosomal dominant condition with complete penetrance and variable expression. It has a prevalence of 1 in 25,000 births and accounts for 5% of cases of craniosynostosis. The disorder occurs in conjunction with a mutation in the FGFR2 gene on chromosome 10q26 [29]. The coronal suture is involved in nearly 95% of cases, but multiple sutures can be affected in this syndrome. There is associated maxillary hypoplasia that leads to a small nasopharynx and narrowed or obliterated anterior nares [2,29]. In addition, hypertelorism, nasal septum deviation, and a "parrot-beak" nose may be present. Brain malformations are uncommon and intelligence is usually normal if patients are managed appropriately (Fig. 13) [29].

Apert syndrome

Apert syndrome is similar to Crouzon syndrome in several ways. Apert syndrome is also an autosomal dominant syndrome that results from a mutation in the FGFR2 gene, but it has a prevalence of only 1 in 160,000 births [29–32]. It is associated with high infant mortality, so the prevalence in the general population is closer to 1 in 2 million [33]. Fused coronal sutures in Apert syndrome is associated with mental retardation and brain malformations [29]. The disorder is characterized by craniosynostosis, midface hypoplasia, and choanal stenosis [2,30]. Other nasal abnormalities include a saddle nose with a bulbous tip and a high-arched palate. Unlike patients affected with Crouzon syndrome, patients who have Apert syndrome have symmetric syndactyly of the hands and feet and other axial skeletal abnormalities.

Pfeiffer syndrome

Pfeiffer syndrome is an autosomal dominant disorder with complete penetrance and variable expression (Fig. 14). The syndrome is related to FGFR1 and FGFR2 mutations, with a prevalence of 1 in 200,000 live births. Craniosynostosis and mental retardation are common features.

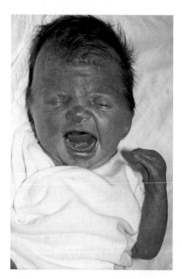

Fig. 13. Apert syndrome.

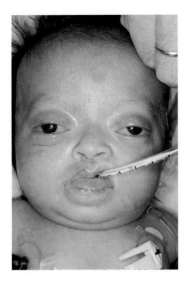

Fig. 14. Pfeiffer syndrome.

The coronal sutures are frequently fused, but the sagittal and lambdoid sutures can also be involved. These patients can have many of the same signs as in Crouzon and Apert syndromes such as a beaked nose, hypertelorism, and midface hypoplasia. In contrast to Apert and Crouzon syndrome, the deformities are less severe and extremity anomalies are present [2,29].

Saethre-Chotzen syndrome

Saethre-Chotzen syndrome is an autosomal dominant disorder with high penetrance and variable expression. The disorder is related to a mutation in the TWIST gene on chromosome 7p21. Craniosynostosis is present in affected patients. Other findings include brachycephaly, a high-arched palate with occasional palatal clefting, a broad depressed nasal bridge, and lacrimal duct stenosis. The frontonasal angle is often depressed. The nose itself may be beaked with a deviated septum [34]. Facial asymmetry was noted in 33% to 52% of cases. Midface hypoplasia occurs but not as commonly as in some of the aforementioned syndromes [2,29,35].

Muenke syndrome

Muenke syndrome is a congenital syndrome similar to the previously defined craniosynostosis syndromes and results from a FGFR3 Pro25Arg mutation. These patients were described to have thimble-like middle phalanges, carpal and tarsal fusions, and brachydactyly. The craniofacial abnormalities are very similar to those displayed in Saethre-Chotzen syndrome [36].

Stickler syndrome

Stickler syndrome is an autosomal dominant syndrome with incomplete penetrance and age-dependent expression. It affects approximately 1 in 10,000 people, making it one of the most common syndromes in the United States [2]. In some families, this genetic defect is localized to the gene COL2A1 on chromosome 12, which codes for type II procollagen, a protein found in vitreous gel and cartilage [37]. Although the disease is primarily characterized by the ophthalmic abnormalities, various orofacial anomalies also develop [38]. The phenotype includes a flattened midface, with a depressed nasal bridge, long philtrum, and shortened, hypoplastic maxilla [39]. Other findings include high-frequency sensorineural hearing loss, bifid uvula, mandibular hypoplasia, and cleft palate. Stickler syndrome is the most common syndrome to be associated with Robin sequence [2,38]. Given its variable expression, the disease, in its mild forms, often goes unrecognized.

Shprintzen syndrome

Shprintzen syndrome (velocardiofacial syndrome) is an autosomal dominant disorder and probably the most common syndrome after Down syndrome. The syndrome occurs as a result of a mutation on 22q11, similar to DiGeorge syndrome. As the name suggests, the syndrome encompasses cardiac, facial, and palatal defects. The main craniofacial abnormalities are clefting of the secondary palate and velopharyngeal incompetence [40]. The nose is prominent, with a broad nasal dorsum and narrow alar base [41]. Immunodeficiency and congenital heart defects may be present with this disorder. The syndrome can often be overlooked because affected patients often appear normal in outward appearance [2].

References

[1] Chang EW, Nguyen C, Lam SM. Emedicine: nose anatomy. Available at: http://www.emedicine.com/ent/topic6.html. Accessed June 26, 2006.
[2] Cummings CW, Haughey BH, Thomas JR, et al. Otolaryngology—head and neck surgery. 4th edition. Philadelphia: Elsevier Mosby; 2005. p. 1001–3, 4031–6, 4099–102.
[3] Gray H. Anatomy of the human body. Philadelphia: Lea & Febiger, 1918; Available at: http://www.bartleby.com.
[4] Netter FH. Atlas of human anatomy. 3rd edition. Teterboro (NJ): ICON Learning Systems; 2003. p. 32–8.
[5] Cutting CB. Secondary cleft lip nasal reconstruction. Cleft Palate Craniofac J 2000;37: 538–41.
[6] Moore CC, MacDonald I, Latham R, et al. Septopalatal protraction for correction of nasal septal deformity in cleft palate infants. Otolaryngol Head Neck Surg 2005;133:949–53.
[7] Lee WT, Koltai PJ. Nasal deformity in neonates and young children. Pediatr Clin North Am 2003;50:459–67.
[8] Wong KS, Lin JL. An underrecognized cause of respiratory distress in a neonate. CMAJ 2006;174(11):1558–9.

[9] Murali H, Hurt H. Nasal molding: a cultural practice causing respiratory distress in a term infant. J Pediatr 2004;144(3):403–4.

[10] Vercruysse J, Wojciechowski M, Koninckx M, et al. Congenital nasal pyriform aperture stenosis: a rare cause of neonatal nasal obstruction. J Pediatr Surg 2006;41:E5–7.

[11] Lee JJ, Bent JP, Ward RF. Congenital nasal pyriform aperture stenosis: non-surgical management and long term analysis. Int J Pediatr Otorhinolaryngol 2001;60:167–71.

[12] Denoyelle F, Ducroz V, Roger G, et al. Nasal dermoid sinus cysts in children. Laryngoscope 1997;107(6):795–800.

[13] Manning S, Bloom D, Perkins J, et al. Diagnostic and surgical challenges in the pediatric skull base. Otolaryngol Clin North Am 2005;38:773–94.

[14] Grunwald L. Bettrage zur kenntnis kongenitaler geschwulste und missbildungen an ohf und nase. Ztsch F Ohrenhik 1910;60:270.

[15] Hanikeri M, Waterhouse N, Kirkpatrick N, et al. The management of midline transcranial nasal dermoid sinus cysts. Br J Plast Surg 2005;58(8):1043–50.

[16] Wardinsky T, Pagon R, Kropp R, et al. Nasal dermoid sinus cyst: association with intracranial extension and multiple malformations. Cleft Palate Craniofac J 1991;28:87–95.

[17] Posnick JC, Bortoluzzi P, Armstrong DC, et al. Intracranial nasal dermoid sinus cysts: computed tomographic scan findings and surgical results. Plast Reconstr Surg 1994;3:745–54.

[18] Fornadley JA, Tami TA. The use of magnetic resonance imaging in the diagnosis of the nasal dermoid sinus-cyst. Otolaryngol Head Neck Surg 1989;101:397–8.

[19] Pollock RA. Surgical approaches to the nasal dermoid cyst. Ann Plast Surg 1983;10: 498–501.

[20] Weiss DD, Robson CD, Mulliken JB. Transnasal endoscopic excision of midline nasal dermoid from the anterior cranial base. Plast Reconstr Surg 1998;101:2119–23.

[21] Trevfik T, Abdulrahman H. Emedicine: choanal atresia. Available at: http://www.emedicine.com/ent/topic330.html. Accessed October 28, 2005.

[22] Hall BD. Choanal atresia in CHARGE syndrome. Available at: http://www.chargesyndrome.org/manual/Choanal.pdf. Accessed 1999.

[23] Behrman R, Kliegman R, Jenson H. Nelson textbook of pediatrics. 17th edition. Philadelphia: Elsevier Science; 2004. p. 1385–8.

[24] Stankiewicz JA. The endoscopic repair or choanal atresia. Otolaryngol Head Neck Surg 1990;103:931–7.

[25] Gross CW, Becker DG. Power instrumentation in endoscopic sinus surgery. Operative Techniques in Otolaryngology Head and Neck Surgery 1996;75:33–8.

[26] Deutsch E, Kaufman M, Eilon A. Transnasal endoscopic management of choanal atresia. Int J Pediatr Otorhinolaryngol 1997;40:19–26.

[27] Brown OE, Pownell P, Manning SC. Choanal atresia: a new anatomic classification and clinical management applications. Laryngoscope 1996;106:97–101.

[28] Crouzon O. Dysostose cranio-raciale hereditaire. Bull Mem Soc Med Hop Paris 1912;33: 545–55.

[29] Ridgway E, Weiner H. Skull deformities. Pediatr Clin North Am 2004;51(2):359–87.

[30] Kabbani H, Raghuveer TS. Craniosynostosis. Am Fam Physician 2004;69(12):2863–70.

[31] Losee JE, Kirschner RE, Whitaker LA, et al. Congenital nasal anomalies: a classification scheme. Plast Reconstr Surg 2004;113(2):676–89.

[32] Rahbar R, Shah P, Mulliken J, et al. The presentation and management of nasal dermoid: a 30 year experience. Arch Otolaryngol Head Neck Surg 2003;129(4):464–71.

[33] Blank CE. Apert's syndrome (a type of acrocephalosyndactyly)—observations on a British series of thirty-nine cases. Ann Hum Genet 1960;24:151–64.

[34] Friedman JM, Hanson JW, Graham CB, et al. Saethre-Chotzen syndrome: a broad and variable pattern of skeletal malformations. J Pediatr 1977;91:929–33.

[35] de Heer IM, de Klein A, van den Ouweland AM, et al. Clinical and genetic analysis of patients with Saethre-Chotzen syndrome. Plastic and Reconstructive Surgery 2005;115(7): 1894–902, discussion 1903–5.

[36] Moloney D, Wall S, Ashworth G, et al. Prevalence of Pro250Arg mutation of fibroblast growth factor receptor in coronal craniosynostosis. Lancet 1997;349:1059–62.
[37] Brown DM, Nichols BE, Weingeist TA, et al. Procollagen II gene mutation in Stickler syndrome. Archives of Ophthalmology 1992;110(11):1589–93.
[38] Rose P, Levy H, Liberfarb R, et al. Sitckler syndrome: clinical characteristics and diagnostic criteria. Am J Med Genet 2005;138A:199–207.
[39] Herrman J, France TD, Spranger JW, et al. The Stickler syndrome (hereditary arthroophthalmopathy). Birth Defects Orig Artic Ser 1975;11(2):76–103.
[40] Losken A, Williams K, Burstein F, et al. Surgical correction of velopharyngeal insufficiency in children with velocardiofacial syndrome. Journal of the American Society of Plastic Surgeons 2006;117(5):1493–8.
[41] Arvystas M, Shprintzen RJ. Craniofacial morphpology in the velo-cardio-facial syndrome. J Craniofac Genet Dev Biol 1984;4:39–45.

ELSEVIER
SAUNDERS

Otolaryngol Clin N Am
40 (2007) 113–140

OTOLARYNGOLOGIC
CLINICS
OF NORTH AMERICA

Congenital Malformations of the Eye and Orbit

Jason R. Guercio, BS[a],*, Lois J. Martyn, MD[b]

[a]University of Pennsylvania School of Medicine, 3450 Hamilton Walk,
Philadelphia, PA 19104, USA
[b]Temple University School of Medicine, Temple University Children's Medicine Center,
Broad and Tioga Streets, Philadelphia, PA 19140, USA

Malformations of the eye, orbit, and ocular adnexa are known to occur in isolation, in combination, or as part of a larger systemic malformation syndrome. Many malformations can severely impair vision, others have only cosmetic significance, and still others cause no symptoms and may go undiscovered or may be noted incidentally on routine eye examination [1]. Congenital anomalies have various causes. The most common causes are defects in genes critical to normal development, but also include aneuploidies, in-utero exposure to exogenous teratogens (ie, drugs or infectious microorganisms), and obstetrical complication (ie, oligohydramnios) [2–4]. Both germline and somatic mutations can cause congenital malformations. Much of the advancement in the field of dysmorphology and in the understanding of congenital malformations in recent years is the result of progress with the genome projects (including the human genome project), which have broadened understanding of the genes implicated in eye and orbit development, and provided a genetic basis for many human developmental eye diseases, including many well-known syndromes with malformed eyes and orbits [5]. Four categories of congenital anomalies have been proposed, including those resulting from (1) single morphogenetic defects, (2) intrauterine mechanical constraint on an otherwise normal embryo or fetus, (3) destruction of a normal structure, and (4) dysplasia, defined as a defect in the differentiation and organization of a tissue. Many of these dysplasias are caused by a single morphogenetic anomaly in development that leads to a subsequent series of defects, defining a sequence or syndrome [2].

* Corresponding author.
E-mail address: guercio@mail.med.upenn.edu (J.R. Guercio).

0030-6665/07/$ - see front matter © 2007 Elsevier Inc. All rights reserved.
doi:10.1016/j.otc.2006.11.013   oto.theclinics.com

Embryology of the human eye

The major structures of the eye are derived from ectoderm, both neural and surface. The sequence of steps that follow have been presented in much greater detail with illustrations elsewhere [6]. The optic pits are formed at 22 days' gestation and then extend outward to form the optic vesicles at 26 to 27 days' gestation. These then contact the overlying surface ectoderm, causing both layers to invaginate. The optic vesicles then form the optic cups at about 4 weeks' gestation, with the inner layer forming the neural (or neurosensory) retina and the outer layer forming the pigmented retina (or pigmented retinal epithelium). The lens placode and lens vesicle then form through a process of invagination and pinching off of surface ecto-derm. This process also contributes to formation of the presumptive cornea [5,7].

The retina begins to differentiate very early in embryogenesis. At 26 days, three to four rows of cells are present, and by 32 to 33 days, five to six rows line the inner layer of the optic cup. Maturation and melanization of the ret-inal pigment epithelium begins posteriorly at the site of the presumptive macula and proceeds peripherally [5,7]. The ganglion cells are produced first, followed by cone photoreceptors, horizontal and amacrine cells, later rod photoreceptors, and finally bipolar cells and Muller cells [8].

Primary vitreous, a highly vascularized gel, develops between weeks 4 and 6, and is then replaced with the avascular secondary vitreous and finally the tertiary vitreous (the suspensory zonules) by the fourth month of gesta-tion [7]. The optic cup, which is connected to the developing forebrain by the optic stalk, contains an inferior and ventral fold, denoted the *embryonic fissure*, through which mesenchymal and vascular tissues, including the hy-aloid artery and a branch of the ophthalmic artery, enter the globe. Closure of this fissure between the fifth and seventh week through cell division and apoptosis is critical to normal iris development. Incomplete closure leads to colobomas of the iris, retina, or choroid [5,7]. The vascular system of the eye and orbit is derived from the primitive internal carotid system, and the primitive dorsal ophthalmic artery supplies the entire eye and orbit at this time [7].

Melanogenesis at optic fissure closure results in vacuolation of the inner layers of the optic stalk to accommodate nerve fibers sent out by differenti-ating retinal neurons. Immigration of retinal ganglion cell axons results in optic nerve formation [5]. Pruning of the initial overproduction of axons re-sults in confirmed connections and the elimination of nonfunctional pro-cesses; approximately 1.2 million active fibers remain with some crossover at the optic chiasm. Myelination of the optic nerve occurs between 5 and 8 months' gestation and proceeds from the geniculate bodies to the globe. Ectopic myelination of the nerve fiber layer within the eye can be seen in some patients as a flat, feathery, glossy white sheen on the surface of the retina (Fig. 1) [7].

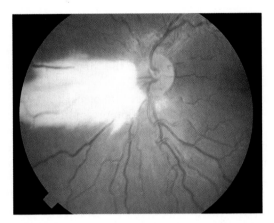

Fig. 1. Myelinated fibers. Feathery white patch of ectopic medullation of retinal nerve fibers.

Cornea and iris form at about 6 weeks' gestation. The first of three waves of mesenchymal cell migrations produces the corneal inner epithelium and the trabecular meshwork, the second results in formation of the corneal stroma, and the third forms the iris stroma. Two anterior chamber structures, the angle and the ciliary body, also develop at approximately 6 weeks' gestation. Lens development is hastened at this point by atrophy of the hyaloid artery and closure of the lumen of the lens vesicle by 7 weeks' gestation [5]. The lens, derived from the lens epithelium and developed by formation of primary and secondary lens fibers, begins to reduce DNA synthesis at its posterior pole, resulting in cell elongation and the development of an organized series of crystallins and other lens proteins [5,7]. Choroid and sclera are formed from condensations of mesenchymal neural crest cells [5].

Extraocular muscles develop from masses of paraxial mesoderm during weeks 4 to 5, with scleral insertion by the second month of gestation. Levator palpebrae superioris is the last striated extraocular muscle to form, occurring during the third month of gestation. The eyelids develop from ectoderm, mesoderm, and, in the case of the tarsus and connective tissue of the eyelid, mesenchymal neural crest cells [7]. These structures begin to differentiate at the sixth week of gestation, fusing at the eighth week. The eyelids begin to separate around the fifth month, beginning nasally and extending temporally, with complete separation by the seventh month [2,7]. The lacrimal glands are formed from epithelial buds arising from the basal epithelial layer of the conjunctiva. Canalization of the lacrimal duct begins at the third month of gestation and is usually completed by the sixth month, but a persistent closure of the lower portion of the duct at birth may result in congenital nasolacrimal duct obstruction. The dilator and sphincter muscles of the iris develop from neuroectoderm between the sixth and eighth months of gestation, and iris vasculature stems from mesoderm [7].

The orbit, which is formed by seven bones, including the maxillary, zygo-matic, frontal, sphenoid, palatine, ethmoid, and lacrimal, undergoes rapid changes in size and shape beginning at 6 months' gestation. The orbital diameter begins to increase rapidly at this time, after transitioning from a previous linear growth curve [7].

Genetic regulation is critical to successful ocular embryogenesis. The two genes that have been described as most important in ocular development are the *PAX6* gene (chromosome 11p13) and the *Rx* gene (chromosome 18). Both genes belong to a large family of factors that are related to the home-odomain region of the *Drosophila* paired protein. Early induction of both genes causes a series of gene activations and depressions which are tanta-mount to normal development of the mature eye. *Rx* and *PAX6* are both expressed in proliferating cells. *PAX6* is also expressed in surface ectoderm of the lens primordia. Mutations of *PAX6* have been shown to lead to anir-idia, congenital cataract, Peter's anomaly, and midline fusion defects. Ab-sence of the gene leads to anophthalmia. *Rx* is associated with retinal proliferation [7]. Other genes that are believed to be involved in ocular development include *FOXC1* and *PITX2* genes, mutations of which have been described in Axenfeld-Rieger syndrome [9–11]. Normal eye anatomy is depicted in Fig. 2.

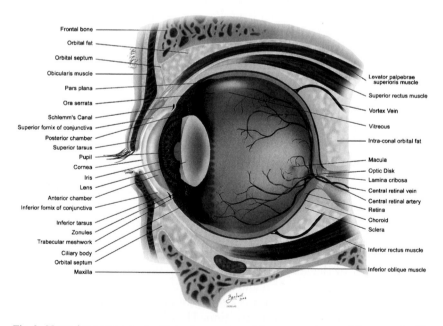

Fig. 2. Normal eye anatomy. Sagittal cut-away view of the gross anatomy of the eye and orbit. (*Illustration by* Adrienne J. Boutwell and Lisa J. Birmingham. © University of Illinois Board of Trustees 2002.)

Congenital abnormalities and syndromes of the eye

Abnormalities of the anterior segment of the eye

Anterior segment dysgenesis

A significant number of congenital ocular anomalies, all of them rare, involve the anterior segment of the eye, which includes the cornea, iris, ciliary body, and lens. The most common of these uncommon disorders is termed the *Axenfeld-Rieger spectrum of anomalies*, which includes several abnormalities, such as posterior embryotoxon (an arcuate white line in the periphery of the cornea), abnormalities of pupillary shape or location, polycoria (full-thickness defects of the iris independent of pupillary defects), and adhesions between the iris and cornea. These ocular abnormalities may coexist with a spectrum of extraocular anomalies as part of an autosomal dominant multisystem congenital disorder that includes facial dysmorphism, redundant periumbilical skin, and anomalies of dentition. Many patients who have Axenfeld-Rieger develop glaucoma, and therefore should be periodically screened for this condition [1].

Peter's anomaly

Children born with a characteristic white opacity of the cornea are classified as having Peter's anomaly. The opacity is usually, but not necessarily, an avascular, central defect that causes a significant visual disturbance. Patients often also exhibit iridocorneal adhesions with or without an anteriorly displaced cataractous lens. Peter's anomaly may be unilateral or bilateral, and patients are predisposed to glaucoma. In the absence of absolute contraindications, surgery for Peter's anomaly, which includes corneal transplantation with or without lens extraction, must proceed at an early age to avoid irreversible amblyopia resulting from visual deprivation in the first weeks of life. An alternative procedure involves the resection of a large section of iris (sector iridectomy) to allow the child to see around the corneal opacity [1].

Peter's anomaly is known to occur in isolation, as part of a larger ocular syndrome such as aniridia or microphthalmia, or as part of a systemic syndromic presentation in Peter's Plus syndrome, involving developmental delay, short stature, and skeletal dysplasia [1].

Peter's anomaly is believed to represent a nonheritable disorder and has been associated with mutations in the *PAX6* gene and the *CYP1B1* gene for congenital glaucoma [1].

Other congenital opacities of the cornea

Several other corneal opacities are congenital in origin. A primary bilateral, gray-white corneal opacification is seen in congenital hereditary endothelial dystrophy (CHED) involving the innermost corneal layer and in congenital hereditary stromal dystrophy (CHSD) involving the middle layer of the cornea. A primary white vascularized opacification of the cornea is characteristic of sclerocornea; focal white opaque lesions suggest corneal dermoid [1]. Although not typically threatening to the visual axis, dermoids of the corneal limbus, which are small white masses that often have hairs growing from them, may cause amblyopia secondary to astigmatism, may cause ocular discomfort, and are seen in Goldenhar syndrome (oculo–auricular–vertebral spectrum). Goldenhar syndrome results from aberrant development of the first or second branchial arch and includes, in addition to epibulbar dermoids, hemifacial microsomia with resultant orbital asymmetry, small ears with skin tags, and vertebral anomalies [1,2].

Corneal clouding may also occur secondary to a host of metabolic storage diseases (although the cornea is often clear at birth), cystinosis, congenital infection, and birth or amniocentesis trauma. Forceps injury to the cornea with rupture of Descemet's membrane may result in corneal clouding caused by edema. A large-appearing, cloudy cornea is a frequent presentation of congenital glaucoma (Fig. 3) [1].

Aniridia

Aniridia is a rare ocular disorder characterized by deficiency of iris tissue, ranging from mild hypoplasia to almost total absence of iris. Associated abnormalities include macular and optic nerve hypoplasia (ONH), cataracts, glaucoma and progressive corneal opacification, attendant vision impairment, and nystagmus (Fig. 4).

Aniridia may occur as a familial autosomal dominant disorder or as a sporadic disorder. It may occur in isolation or in association with several systemic abnormalities. In particular, sporadic aniridia is associated with Wilm's tumor, and often also with genitourinary abnormalities and mental retardation (WAGR), attributed to mutation of the *PAX6* gene on chromosome 11p13 [12].

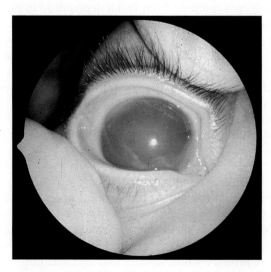

Fig. 3. Generalized corneal clouding. An important sign of congenital glaucoma.

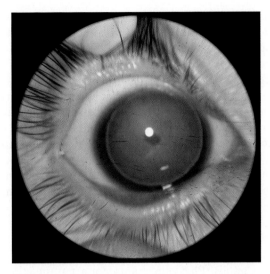

Fig. 4. Aniridia. Note rudimentary iris rim and anterior polar cataract.

Persistent pupillary membranes

Incomplete resorption of the normal intrauterine pupillary membrane rarely results in visual disturbance and is more frequently an incidental finding, with small strands projecting freely from the iris into the anterior chamber, or longer strands, even fine webs, spanning the pupil (Fig. 5). Typically, lysis of the strands results from physiologic pupillary constriction and dilation, but pharmacologic dilation may be needed in refractory cases. Surgery is usually indicated only if substantial strands or bands attach to the lens, causing miosis or cataract. Prompt referral to an ophthalmologist is

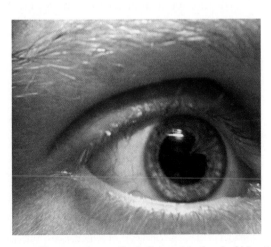

Fig. 5. Persistent pupillary membrane. Pupil distorted by band of iris attached to lens.

indicated if the persistent pupillary strands obstruct the red reflex [1]. Rarely, patent vessels within pupillary membrane remnants can rupture, causing spontaneous hyphema.

Congenital cysts of the margin of the pupil

Originating in the posterior pigmented epithelium of the iris at the pupillary margin, these bead-like cysts cause the edge of the pupil to appear irregular and impart a brownish appearance which is easily seen when checking for the presence of the red reflex. Because these cysts uncommonly involve the visual axis, referral to an ophthalmologist is rarely indicated. Congenital cysts of the pupil margin typically disappear over time, making surgical removal unnecessary. Pharmacologic dilation of the pupil may be used in refractory cases or cases involving the visual axis [1].

Physiologic anisocoria

About a quarter of the population has a size discrepancy of up to 2 mm between the two pupils. Physiologic anisocoria requires that the pupils be round, centrally located, and briskly reactive. If the anisocoria is physiologic, as in most cases, the proportional discrepancy in size will remain relatively constant in all light conditions [1].

Congenital cataract

Congenital cataract occurs in 1:4000 to 1:10,000 newborns (Fig. 6). It may be unilateral or bilateral, an isolated finding, or part of an extensive spectrum of congenital disorders, both heritable and nonheritable, involving chromosomal aberrations; multisystem genetic syndromes; congenital metabolic derangements such as galactosemia; congenital infections; or congenital ocular malformation syndromes such as Peter's anomaly or aniridia. It is a rare result of birth trauma or amniocentesis injury [1].

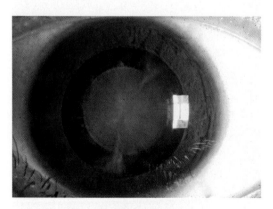

Fig. 6. Congenital cataract. Dense opacification of lens nucleus, sufficient to cause visual deprivation.

By definition, any lens opacity is considered a cataract. Cataracts that do not involve the visual axis may be visually insignificant. Even small central cataracts (<3 mm) may become visually insignificant with the instillation of an accommodation-sparing dilating drop with or without patching of the unaffected eye. Cataracts are described with respect to the part of the lens that is involved. Anterior opacities (anterior polar) include dot anterior polar cataract, anterior lenticonus often associated with Alport syndrome (caused by a defect of collagen and characterized by renal and, less commonly, cochlear anomalies), anterior pyramidal cataract, anterior subcapsular cataract, and anterior capsular opacity associated with persistent pupillary membrane strands. Posterior opacities include posterior polar cataract, posterior lenticonus, and posterior subcapsular cataract (commonly seen in iritis). Cataracts within the lens include nuclear cataract and lamellar cataract, the latter of which involves individual layers of the interior of the lens. Many genes are responsible for the varying presentations of congenital cataract; autosomal dominant, autosomal recessive, and X-linked recessive transmissions occur [1].

Treatment for visually significant congenital cataracts should be initiated immediately after detection (usually by the pediatrician's careful examination of the red reflex, which will appear partially or completely obscured, depending on the size and location of the cataract). Prompt referral to an ophthalmologist is critical for any abnormality of the red reflex, including asymmetry between the eyes and the presence of a white or dark reflex, to establish the diagnosis of congenital cataract or other ocular abnormality and to guide treatment. Urgent referral must be made if congenital cataract is suspected in the first year of life, particularly in the first 6 weeks to 3 months. Although response to treatment diminishes with age, children aged up to 9 to 11 years who have congenital cataract may benefit from treatment [1].

Treatment of the visually significant cataract that is not amenable to pupillary dilation and patching involves removal of the cataractous lens as soon as possible to avoid irreversible failure of visual development resulting from lack of visual input to the affected eye or eyes. The resultant surgical aphakia is then corrected with glasses, contact lenses, or an intraocular lens implant (IOL) at surgery. Intraocular lens insertion for children aged 2 years and older is becoming increasingly accepted in the absence of contraindications such as iritis [1]. IOL implantation in infants can yield poor results [13]. Patching of the phakic eye is a critical treatment component in unilateral congenital cataract [1].

Persistent hyperplastic primary vitreous

Lens development in the embryo is hastened between weeks 6 and 7 of gestation by atrophy of the hyaloid artery, which runs from the optic nerve head to the posterior pole of the lens, and by closure of the lumen of the lens vesicle [1,5]. Failure of resorption of this fetal vasculature leads to a vascularized membrane or stalk that may extend, completely or incompletely, from the disc to the back of the lens, denoted persistent hyperplastic primary vitreous (PHPV). Associated findings, occurring singly or in combination, are microphthalmia, glaucoma, miosis with inability to pharmacologically dilate the pupil, shallow anterior chamber caused by forward bulging of the iris, and contracted ciliary processes that are drawn in toward the pupil. The cause of this anomaly, which is not considered heritable and may be found as an isolated defect or in conjunction with other ocular malformations, is unknown. Rare cases of bilateral PHPV are commonly associated with congenital systemic malformation syndromes. Before the advent of modern diagnostic and therapeutic techniques, visual prognosis with PHPV was poor. Except in the case of retinal scarring or detachment, visual prognosis can be good with early diagnosis and prompt intervention [1].

Anophthalmia, microphthalmia, and colobomata of the iris and retina

With the exception of cyclopia (Fig. 7), anophthalmia, or total absence of the eye, is the most severe ocular abnormality [14]. It represents a developmental-field defect in Pfeifer's diacephalic region, which is subject to some of the most severe craniofacial malformations, including cleft lip, palate, and nose; clefts of the Tessier-type; and anophthalmia, microphthalmia (axial length of the eye shorter than normal) (Fig. 8), and cryptophthalmos

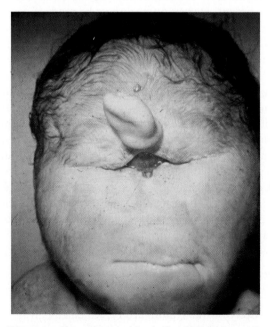

Fig. 7. Cyclopia. Extreme malformation resulting in fused bilobed central eye and proboscis.

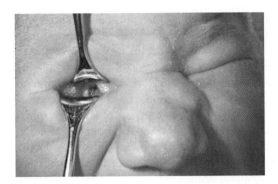

Fig. 8. Microphthalmia. Small eye and short palpebral fissure in infant with trisomy 13.

(congenital absence of the eyelid). Anophthalmia, microphthalmia, and cryptophthalmos are morphogenetically related [4,14]. Anophthalmia and microphthalmia are frequently found in conjunction with hypertelorism and hemifacial microsomia. They were also recently associated with congenital defects of the limb and musculoskeletal systems; other defects of the eye; defects of the ear, face, and neck; and specifically trisomy 18, trisomy 13, other chromosomal abnormalities, amnion rupture sequence, osteogenesis imperfecta, Aicardi syndrome, CHARGE syndrome, Cornelia de Lange syndrome, dwarfism, Goltz syndrome, Meckel-Gruber syndrome, Seckel syndrome, septo-optic dysplasia, short rib–polydactyly dysplasia syndrome, and Werdnig-Hoffmann disease [14]. A large population study of the epidemiology of anophthalmia and microphthalmia in Hawaii recently reported a combined rate of 3.21 per 10,000 live births, an anophthalmia rate of 3.01 per 100,000 live births, a microphthalmia rate of 2.84 per 10,000 live births, and an association with low birth weight and earlier gestational age [15].

Anophthalmia, whether unilateral or bilateral, is always accompanied by hypoplasia of the associated orbits, because the eye normally stimulates orbital growth during development of the midface during childhood [14]. Microphthalmia, if very severe, may have a similar result [1]. If unilateral, facial asymmetry invariably results, with hypoplasia of the midface, a canted occlusal plane, and a short ascending ramus of the mandible. Therefore, especially in unilateral cases of anophthalmia and microphthalmia, orbital growth must be induced using orbital implants of progressively increasing size throughout childhood. The judicious use of self-inflating expanders, most recently of methacrylate-N-vinylpyrrolidone, has been shown to achieve a long-lasting, aesthetically pleasing, physiologic cosmetic result [14].

Microphthalmia may or may not be visually significant, depending on its degree. It may exist with a normal or small cornea (microcornea). Nanophthalmia, a rare form of bilateral microphthalmia, is an autosomal dominant disorder with thick sclera that predisposes patients to spontaneous retinal detachments secondary to subretinal fluid. It is commonly associated with congenital cataract (often nuclear or PHPV) and coloboma, the latter likely the primary cause of microphthalmia. Microphthalmia and coloboma may follow autosomal dominant or autosomal recessive inheritance patterns [1].

Coloboma, or congenital absence of a portion of the tissue of the eye, represents a failure of fusion of the embryonic fissure between the fifth and seventh week of gestation by cell division and apoptosis, leading to defects of the iris, ciliary body, choroid, retina, or optic nerve (Fig. 9) [5,7]. It can appear as an isolated finding or as part of a multisystem syndrome, most frequently as part of the CHARGE (Coloboma of the eye, Heart defects, Atresia of the choanae, Retarded growth and development, Genital hypoplasia, and Ear anomalies with or without deafness) syndrome and in patients who have chromosomal disorders.

Coloboma of the optic nerve may be visually insignificant, with benign enlargement of the optic disc and cup, or may involve the inferior disc with pigmentary disruption and visual loss. It may also extend into the subjacent retina, with failure of the retinal pigment epithelium (RPE) to fuse coupled with absence of the choroid in the affected portion, revealing the underlying sclera on funduscopic examination. Defective retina within the coloboma itself is prone to retinal detachment. If large, retinal coloboma may involve the macula, fovea, and optic nerve simultaneously, with a uniformly poor visual result. In some cases, coloboma may involve only the iris, resulting in a keyhole-shaped pupil of no visual significance, unless the superior pupillary edge is drawn down into the central visual axis [1].

Abnormalities of the optic nerve

Optic nerve hypoplasia

ONH, characterized by a small underdeveloped optic nerve (Fig. 10), may be unilateral or bilateral, and may occur in isolation or with various congenital anomalies of the central nervous system (less common in unilateral cases) and pituitary axis, more commonly known as septo-optic dysplasia. When septo-optic dysplasia occurs in combination with characteristic facies, open anterior fontanelle, and other anomalies of the cerebral midline, the term *de Morsier syndrome* is used, although it is a common practice to use the two terms interchangeably. Mild cases of ONH may be visually insignificant and either escape detection or be seen only on funduscopic examination. More severe cases can show marked deficiency of nervehead tissue, disc pallor, abnormal vessel branching off of the disc, and a "double-ring" sign, reflecting the rim and part of the interior of the scleral canal that an optic nerve of normal size would have otherwise occupied [1].

Vision impairment of ONH ranges from various visual field defects and subnormal acuity to blindness, often with attendant nystagmus and strabismus. Hypothalamic or pituitary involvement in septo-optic dysplasia can cause various endocrine defects, such as growth hormone or thyroid deficiency. MRI of the brain is recommended in suspected cases to identify pituitary, hypothalamic, and cortical pathology; defects of the corpus callosum

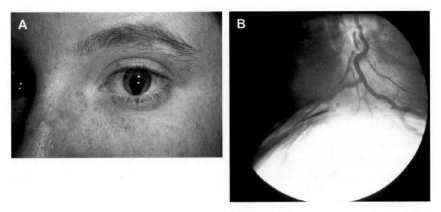

Fig. 9. Colobomata. Wedge-shaped defects of iris (*A*) and fundus (*B*) caused by malclosure of the embryonic fissure.

and septum pellucidum may also be identified. Endocrine evaluation is also advised. In the case of unilateral ONH, patching of the unaffected eye may help minimize amblyopia [1].

ONH has been associated with mutations in the *HESX1* homeobox gene [1]. Effects of fetal alcohol syndrome have been shown to result in hypoplasia of the optic nerve head in 48% of affected infants [16].

Morning glory disc

Morning glory disc, an almost universally unilateral condition, is characterized by the presence of an enlarged optic nerve, retinal vessels arranged in

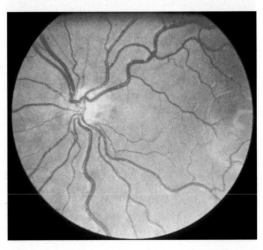

Fig. 10. Optic nerve hypoplasia. Note small deficient nerve, tortuous vessels, and exposed scleral ring.

a spoke-like pattern, and a glial tuft overlying the optic cup. This anomaly may represent a coloboma of the optic disc. On CT or ultrasound, morning glory disc appears as an enlarged, funnel-shaped optic nerve as it enters the globe. Mild to severe vision impairment may be present. In some cases, patching of the unaffected eye may be useful to minimize amblyopia. In rare cases, morning glory anomaly may signify a basal encephalocele, especially with a concomitant notch of the central lower lip [1].

Normal optic nerve variants

Several normal variant optic nerve configurations exist, none of which is associated with decreased vision in the affected eyes. One anomaly involves peripapillary pigmentation, in which the head of the optic nerve is surrounded by a ring of hyperpigmented tissue. When this defect exists on the disc's temporal side, as is more commonly the case in myopia, it is referred to as a *temporal crescent* (Fig. 11). Peripapillary hypopigmentation may represent an area of retinochoroidal atrophy. Another developmental variant involves tilting of the optic disc, most commonly, but not necessarily, secondary to the increased globe length seen in myopia. In these cases, the disc appears slanted on funduscopic examination, with the nasal portion of the nerve more prominent than the temporal, which may make assessment of the optic nerve cup size difficult.

A third variant commonly seen in childhood is physiologic cupping of the optic nerve. This defect is most commonly bilateral and symmetric, but may be unilateral or asymmetric and is believed to have autosomal dominant inheritance when the parents are affected. The cup/disc ratio may be as high as

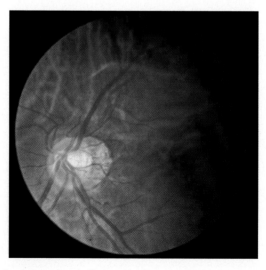

Fig. 11. Temporal crescent. Area of exposed sclera temporal to disc margin is a common developmental variant.

0.8, and the physiologic cup will typically display very sharp edges with some splaying of the vessels as they exit the cup. Glaucoma must be ruled out in a child who presents with a high cup/disc ratio, and referral to an ophthalmologist is advised.

A fourth variant, most commonly seen in hyperopic children, is pseudo-papilledema, in which the optic nerve head appears swollen although no true edema or evidence of increased intracranial pressure is present. The edges of the disc may be blurry and the disc may appear elevated, but other features of true papilledema, such as disc hyperemia, absence of spontaneous venous pulsations, and small hemorrhages or exudates of the nerve fiber layer, will be absent. Pseudopapilledema may be the result of buried drusen, which may be identifiable only with imaging studies such as CT or ultrasound. Rarely, these may be associated with visual field defects or subretinal fluid leakage [1].

Congenital abnormalities and syndromes of the orbit and other periocular tissues

Abnormalities of distance between the eyes and orbits

It is important to distinguish between normal and abnormal to clinically assess the many abnormalities of the orbit and periocular tissues. A substantial number of congenital malformations have an abnormal distance between the eyes as a cardinal feature. The interorbital distance, which is the shortest distance between the medial orbital walls, increases with age, and can be most accurately assessed using bony interorbital distances from roentgenograms (Waters' [half-axial] projection or posteroanterior cephalograms) or CT.

In everyday practice, the following landmarks should be part of any clinical examination when a congenital abnormality of the orbit or other periocular tissue is suspected: interpupillary distance (IPD), inner intercanthal distance (ICD), outer intercanthal distance (OCD), and horizontal palpebral length, which can all then be compared with normal values (Fig. 12) [2]. Several routine methods have been described for assessing interocular distance [17–19]. Notation of whether the palpebral fissures are upslanting or down-slanting is also important, because these anomalies are common in congenital syndromes, such as the upward-slanting palpebral fissures in Down syndrome.

Hypotelorism

Hypotelorism is defined as a decreased distance between the medial orbital walls (interorbital distance), with abnormally small inner and outer canthal distances (Fig. 13) [1,2]. Hypotelorism has been described in more than 60 syndromes and can be the result of a skull malformation or a failure in brain development. For example, trigonocephaly, a rare craniosynostosis

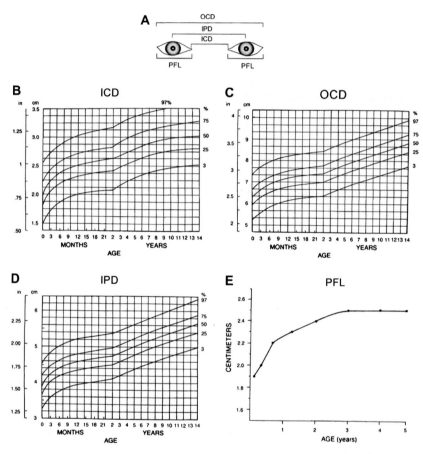

Fig. 12. (*A*) Schematic representation of measurements involved in the evaluation of the orbital region. (*B*) ICD measurements according to the age. (*C*) OCD measurements according to the age. (*D*) IPD measurements according to the age. (*E*) Normal PFL measurements according to the age. OCD, outer canthal distance; ICD, inner canthal distance; IPD, interpupillary distance; PFL, palpebral fissure length. (*From* Dollfus H, Verloes A. Dysmorphology and the orbital region: a practical clinical approach. Surv Ophthalmol 2004;49(6):547–61; with permission.)

caused by premature closure of the metopic sutures, results in hypotelorism, a triangular skull, and a prominent frontal protuberance [20].

Hypotelorism may be seen associated with holoprosencephaly, a rare major brain malformation that results from abnormal cleavage and morphogenesis during the third week of fetal development [21]. It may be caused by environmental or maternal factors, aneuploidy, or defects in single genes. Related craniofacial abnormalities occur on a spectrum from a single median orbit with fused globes (cyclopia) with an overhanging proboscis to a much milder anomaly that includes a single maxillary incisor with hypotelorism [2].

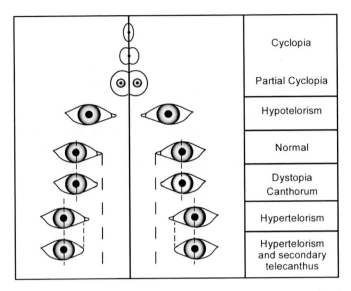

		Cyclopia
		Partial Cyclopia
		Hypotelorism
		Normal
		Dystopia Canthorum
		Hypertelorism
		Hypertelorism and secondary telecanthus

Fig. 13. Schematic representation of abnormal distances between the eyes ranging from cyclopia (fused eyes and orbits) to major hypertelorism with secondary telecanthus. (*From* Dollfus H, Verloes A. Dysmorphology and the orbital region: a practical clinical approach. Surv Ophthalmol 2004;49(6):547–61; with permission.)

Hypertelorism

Hypertelorism is defined as an increased distance between the medial orbital walls (interorbital distance), with abnormally large inner and outer canthal distances (but notably not of the inner canthi only) (see Fig. 13) [1,2]. Clinically, the interpupillary distance is increased. Hypertelorism may coexist with a cribriform plate defect with or without an anterior encephalocele. Incorrect diagnoses of hypertelorism are often the result of a flat nasal bridge, epicanthal folds, exotropia, widely spaced eyebrows, narrow palpebral fissures, and isolated dystopia canthorum. Hypertelorism has been described in more than 550 disorders [2].

Three potential mechanisms of hypertelorism have been advanced, each of which offers a plausible explanation for its syndromic significance. The first includes early ossification of the lesser wings of the sphenoid, fixing the orbits in the fetal position (from a widely divergent 180° during early development to 70° at birth, both greater than the normal 68° angle seen in adulthood). The second describes developmental failure of the nasal capsule, allowing the primitive brain vesicle to protrude into this space, thereby arresting evolution of the position of the eyes, as can be seen in frontal encephalocele [22]. The third potential mechanism of hypertelorism is a proposed skull base developmental disturbance, as can be seen in craniosynostosis syndromes such as Apert's and Crouzon syndromes, or in midfacial malformations such as frontonasal dysplasia or craniofacial dysplasia [2,23,24].

Telecanthus and dystopia canthorum

Telecanthus refers to a large distance between the two medial canthi compared with the interorbital distance (see Fig. 13). The formal definition of telecanthus is a Mustardé ratio (ICD/IPD) greater than 0.55 [25]. Telecanthus is suspected when the lower lid puncta lie lateral to the medial edge of the iris in straight-ahead gaze (termed *dystopia canthorum*) (see Fig. 13). The normal position of the punctum is medial to the medial iris edge [1,2]. Telecanthus can be primary, in which an increased ICD exists with a normal IPD and OCD, or secondary, in which an increased ICD exists with an increased OCD (ocular hypertelorism) [2].

Telecanthus is a common feature in many congenital syndromes; dystopia canthorum can be seen in Waardenburg syndrome type 1, an autosomal dominant syndrome with a broad nasal root, poliosis (often a white forelock), heterochromia irides, and sensorineural hearing loss [26,27]. Dystopia canthorum is not present in Waardenburg syndrome type 2 [2].

Abnormalities of the eyes in relation to their respective orbits

Prominent eyes

Prominent eyes refer to either a protrusion of normal globes, an increased volume of the globes, or a combination of the two. The former is denoted proptosis (or exophthalmos), and can be the result of forward displacement of the normal globe beyond the normal orbital margin or as a result of a normal globe in the setting of reduced orbital depth (shallow orbit). Pseudoproptosis refers to enlargement of the eye, often caused by buphthalmos (congenital glaucoma) or high-degree myopia, causing the appearance of prominent eyes in the context of normal orbits [2].

Craniosynostosis syndromes, such as the aforementioned Apert and Crouzon syndromes, result in prominent eyes caused by underdevelopment of the orbital ridges and midfacial bones, which reduces the orbital volume.

Midfacial retrusion or hypoplasia in general is associated with prominent eyes, and both frequently coexist as part of several congenital syndromes. The autosomal dominant Stickler syndrome, for example, is characterized by a variable presentation that can include midfacial hypoplasia, prominent eyes, cleft palate, micrognathia, sensorineural deafness with high tone loss, and spondyloepiphyseal dysplasia. Eye prominence in Stickler syndrome is heightened by high-degree myopia and abnormalities of vitreous gel architecture [28]. Midfacial hypoplasia is also a prominent feature of Schinzel-Giedion syndrome, which, in addition to prominent eyes, is characterized by degeneration of the central nervous system; skeletal, cardiac, and renal anomalies; bitemporal narrowing; and a figure-eight appearance of the midface caused by the presence of a deep groove under the eyes [29].

Sunken eyes

Sunken eyes are a rare feature in dysmorphology, and are commonly caused by a defect in orbital development, in which the orbital ridges and walls are overly prominent, but may also result from insufficient development of the globes or loss of fatty tissue within the orbit [2]. For example, Cockayne syndrome is an autosomal recessive premature aging disorder of DNA repair characterized by sunken eyes secondary to melting of orbital fat, and has a variable presentation that may include sensorineural hearing loss, cataracts, pigmentary retinopathy, cutaneous photosensitivity, and dental caries [30].

Abnormalities of the size, shape, and symmetry of the orbits

An abnormal shape or size of one or both orbits may result from a primary developmental defect or as a result of a primary intraorbital process that results in aberrant orbital growth in utero or postnatally. A primary orbital process that can result in abnormalities of orbital shape is craniosynostosis, a cardinal feature of several congenital syndromes involving the skull bones that contribute to formation of the orbit [2].

Increased size of the orbit, typically unilateral and therefore also resulting in orbital asymmetry, is a frequent consequence of an intraorbital mass such as an encephalocele, tumor, or cystic eye. A small orbit, either unilateral or bilateral, frequently coexists with microphthalmia or anophthalmia, wherein the affected orbit fails to grow because of a lack of normal interaction between the growing eye and the orbital walls.

Asymmetry of the orbits is a frequent feature of congenital syndromes affecting the eye and/or orbit, including the previously mentioned Goldenhar syndrome (oculoauriculovertebral spectrum), whose orbital asymmetry is the result of hemifacial microsomia [1,2]. Congenital tumors and sphenoid wing dysplasia, such as those seen in neurofibromatosis type 1, and congenital orbital hamartomas, such as those occurring in Proteus syndrome, may also result in orbital asymmetry [2,31].

Abnormalities of the eyelids

Cryptophthalmos

Cryptophthalmos, a rare congenital malformation, refers to complete failure of development of the eyelids, with skin continuity from the forehead to the cheek. It is a common feature of Fraser syndrome, a rare autosomal recessive disorder associated with hypoplastic genitalia, laryngeal stenosis, and renal anomalies [2].

Ablepharon

Ablepharon is an exceedingly rare condition that describes a total absence of the eyelids and is the defining feature of the autosomal recessive ablepharon-macrostomia syndrome, also associated with auricular deformity, nasal alar deformity, absence of lanugo hair, ichthyotic skin, ambiguous genitalia, and absence of the zygomatic arches [32].

Epicanthus

Epicanthus describes a common, mild eyelid anomaly with rare visual or syndromic significance. Four types of abnormal epicanthal folds exist: epicanthus inversus, epicanthus tarsalis, epicanthus palpebralis, and epicanthus supraciliaris [33]. Epicanthus inversus, a redundant fold arising from the lower lid, is the only epicanthal fold with syndromic significance, and is seen in blepharophimosis [1]. Epicanthus tarsalis is typical of East Asians with normal facies. Along with epicanthus palpebralis, a fold arising from the nasal root and directed toward the medial upper eyelids is the most common type seen [2]. Epicanthus supraciliaris has its origin in the upper eyelid close to the eyebrows [1].

Epiblepharon

Epiblepharon refers to a common mild congenital malformation involving a redundant skin fold below the lid margin of one or both eyelids, resulting in direction of the eyelashes toward the cornea, occasionally causing trichiasis and corneal damage. It is more common in Asians of the Far East. With advancing age, the eyelashes tend to assume a more normal position. The upper eyelid may be involved in rare instances [1].

Congenital ptosis (congenital blepharoptosis)

Congenital ptosis (congenital blepharoptosis), defined as a drooping of the upper eyelid, may be unilateral or bilateral, with more severe forms involving hypoplasia of the levator palpebrae superioris muscle or tendon with a minimal or absent eyelid crease [1,2]. Symptoms occur on a spectrum, from no visual or cosmetic disturbance with mild ptosis, to visual impairment resulting in compensatory positioning of the head, difficulty in daily activities, and significant cosmetic deformity with severe ptosis. If the lower margin of the upper eyelid falls to or below the center of the pupil, vision may be affected. This often causes children to adopt a chin-up posture for viewing objects straight ahead, with resultant difficulty ambulating, or they may arch their eyebrows using forehead muscles to partially elevate their eyelids. Early surgical correction of ptosis is often indicated to prevent amblyopia, but in less severe cases surgery may be deferred to affect a more favorable outcome. Some children who have congenital ptosis may exhibit Marcus Gunn jaw winking, in which jaw movement results in simultaneous elevation of the upper eyelid [1].

Congenital ptosis may be associated with several congenital syndromes (although it is rarely the hallmark), especially those involving disorders of eye movement, such as congenital fibrosis of the extraocular muscles. It is commonly present in Smith-Lemli-Opitz syndrome, associated with a defect in cholesterol biosynthesis, and Noonan syndrome, an autosomal dominant condition characterized by congenital heart disease, short stature, abnormal facies, and the somatic features of Turner syndrome [34,35]. It can be seen as a major feature of Saethre-Chotzen syndrome, an autosomal dominant craniosynostosis syndrome with minor limb anomalies and characteristic facies mapped to chromosome 7p [36]. It is also a common feature of Cornelia de Lange syndrome, a rare multisystem malformation disorder with characteristic facial features, growth and cognitive retardation, and abnormalities of the limbs, gastrointestinal system, respiratory system, genitourinary system, auditory and ocular systems, kidneys, heart, blood cells, and hair [37].

Blepharophimosis

Blepharophimosis is morphologically defined as reduction of both the horizontal and vertical dimensions of the palpebral fissure, and can occur in isolation or as part of a number of congenital syndromes. This should not be confused with vertical narrowing of the palpebral fissure due to ptosis or with reduction of horizontal fissure length due to curvature of the palpebral rim; the latter can be commonly seen in Down syndrome and Prader-Willi syndrome [2].

Blepharophimosis, ptosis, and epicanthus inversus coexist in a syndrome by the same name (BPES), which is transmitted in an autosomal dominant fashion and has been mapped to chromosome 3q22–23 [1,2]. This syndrome may also be associated with strabismus [1]. It exists in two forms: BPES type I and BPES type II. BPES type I is characterized by infertility in affected females [38]. Ohdo syndrome is a sporadic syndrome that incorporates blepharophimosis, ptosis, dental hypoplasia, partial deafness, and mental retardation [39]. Blepharophimosis can also be seen in several aneuploidies, such as in association with ptosis in chromosome 3p deletion [40]. Fetal alcohol effects are among the most common causes of blepharophimosis [16].

Ectropion and euryblepharon

Ectropion refers to the eversion of the entire length of the lower eyelid. It can result in lagophthalmos and exposure keratopathy if left untreated. It is typically seen as a consequence of aging, but may also be seen as a congenital anomaly, as in several autosomal recessive skin disorders such as congenital cutis laxa with looseness of the lid or as cicatricial ectropion in harlequin ichthyosis. It has also been associated with macrostomia, ectropion, atrophic skin hypertrichosis syndrome, and blepharocheilodontic syndrome [2].

Euryblepharon is a congenital defect of increased horizontal length of the eyelids of unknown origin. The increased horizontal length of the palpebral fissure coupled with decreased eyelid skin in the vertical dimension causes the lateral portion of the eyelid to become everted (lateral ectropion). It is typically, but not necessarily, symmetric, and more commonly involves the lower eyelids. It may be seen in isolation, or with a host of other ocular anomalies, such as displacement of the proximal lacrimal drainage system, a double row of meibomian gland orifices, telecanthus, and strabismus. As is the case with ectropion, in severe cases it may result in lagophthalmos and exposure keratopathy [41]. It is characteristic of Kabuki make-up syndrome, a constellation that also includes mental and growth retardation, large and protruding ears, and characteristic facies [42].

Coloboma of the eyelid

Congenital notching of the upper or lower eyelid margin is referred to as eyelid coloboma. It is usually triangular with the base at the lid margin and varies from a small notch to a major defect when present on the lower eyelid [2]. It is more commonly medial or central with a rectangular shape when it is present in the upper eyelid, and is commonly associated with lid-to-globe attachments. Although upper lid coloboma does not usually have a negative impact on vision; colobomata of the lower eyelid may result in ulceration or desiccation of the inferior cornea [1]. The exact cause of eyelid coloboma is unknown, although intrauterine factors are believed to contribute [2].

Coloboma of the eyelids can be seen in isolation or as part of congenital malformation syndromes. It has been described as a result of the amnion rupture sequence caused by mechanical disruption [43]. Upper eyelid colobomas are commonly found in the previously mentioned Goldenhar syndrome (oculoauricularvertebral spectrum) [1,2]. Lower lid colobomas, especially with a typical downsweeping with an upsweep to the lateral canthus and an absence of the lower eyelashes, are typical of autosomal dominant Treacher Collins syndrome (mandibulofacial dysostosis); this is a syndrome of aberrant development of the first branchial arch also characterized by auditory anomalies with bilateral conductive hearing loss, hypoplasia of the facial bones, cleft palate, and down-slanting palpebral fissures [2,44]. A "wave shape" of the palpebral fissure is characteristic of the Cohen syndrome, with microcephaly; developmental delay; slim, tapering extremities with truncal obesity; hypotonia; joint laxity; neutropenia; retinal degeneration or myopia; and characteristic facies [45].

Ankyloblepharon (ankyloblepharon filiforme adnatum)

Ankyloblepharon (ankyloblepharon filiforme adnatum) is a rare defect, typically seen in isolation, characterized by a persistent connection between the ciliary edges of the upper and lower eyelid margins [46]. Ankyloblepharon does not usually affect vision, because the connections tend to be small, but larger connections may occur with partial or full obstruction of vision. Surgical excision is curative [1].

Ankyloblepharon has been described in the autosomal dominant Hay-Wells syndrome with ectodermal dysplasia and cleft lip or palate, and in neonates who have Edwards syndrome [46,47].

Abnormalities of the eyelashes and eyebrows

Abnormalities of the eyelashes and eyebrows are present in several congenital syndromes.

Rubinstein-Taybi syndrome is associated with prominent eyelashes; heavy, arched eyebrows; and down-slanting palpebral fissures, in addition to mental retardation and skeletal deformities [48]. Cornelia de Lange syndrome is associated with long, curly eyelashes with synophrys, defined as eyebrows extending to the midline [2]. Trichomegaly, or long eyelashes, is associated with the congenitally acquired Oliver-McHarlane syndrome, in association with retinal dystrophy, mental retardation, and prenatal onset growth failure [49]. Ectrodactyly ectodermal dysplasia clefting syndrome is a condition with autosomal dominant transmission that involves sparse eyebrows and eyelashes in addition to sparse or absent hair, brittle nails, dental anomalies, and split hands (ectrodactyly) [50]. A double row of eyelashes (distichiasis) is a central feature of lymphedema-distichiasis syndrome, which has recently been mapped to chromosome 16q24.3 [51].

Genes in developmental eye disease

In recent decades, knowledge of congenital anomalies of the eye and orbit has been advanced through inquiry into the genetic basis of developmental eye disease. Several specific gene families and individual genes have been identified as responsible for different eye and orbit abnormalities and syndromes (Table 1). Many systemic syndromes, although apparently traced to mutations at a specific gene locus, exhibit broad phenotypic heterogeneity. Mutations at different loci also have been shown to produce similar phenotypes. These facts suggest that many of these genes may affect the same developmental pathway [5].

Recently, anomalies of the anterior segment have been linked to a group of genes, including *PAX6*, *PITX2*, *PITX3*, and *FKHL7*, all of which are transcriptional regulators with highly conserved motifs that translate into specific DNA-binding domains. Each of these genes exhibits extraocular expression; however, the phenotype seems to be limited to the eye. Each gene has been found to be associated with haploinsufficiency, suggesting a stoichiometric relationship between resultant proteins and partner molecules. In addition, an excess of *PAX6* has also been found to be deleterious. *PAX6* is associated with gene product truncation, whereas *PITX2*, *PITX3*, and *FKHL7* are associated with loss of function or missense mutations [5].

Cone–rod dystrophies have been linked to mutations in *CRX*, *RETGC1*, *PRPH*, and *RPE65*, all of which are specifically involved in retinal development and maintenance. *CRX* is a photoreceptor transcriptional regulator, *RETGC1* is a GMP regulator in phototransduction, *PRPH* (peripherin) is a photoreceptor outer segment component, and *RPE65* is an RPE-specific protein of unknown function. Disease-causing mutations of these genes

Table 1
Human developmental eye disease: genes identified

Primary disease	Gene	Major eye phenotype	Variable associated anomalies: eye and other	Other primary eye phenotypes involving the same gene
Eye specific phenotypes Aniridia	*PAX6*	Absence or hypoplasia of the iris	Cataract, glaucoma, corneal abnormalities nystagmus	Peter's anomaly with posterior embryotoxon, iris hypoplasia, congenital cataract, anterior keratitis, isolated foveal hypoplasia
Rieger's syndrome	*PITX2* (=*RIEG1*)	Anterior segment abnormalities strongly overlapping with *FKHL7* mutant phenotype	Glaucoma, tooth anomalies, umbilical stump abnormalities	Iris hypoplasia, iridogoniodysgenesis
Anterior segment mesodermal dysgenesis	*PITX3*	Corneal opacities, with or without iris adhesions, variable severity cataracts	Optic nerve abnormalities	Congenital cataract
Anterior segment anomaly with glaucoma	*FKHL7*	Abnormal iridocorneal angle differentiation (goniodysgenesis), iris stromal hypoplasia, and elevated intraocular pressure/glaucoma	Iris hypoplasia, posterior embryotoxon	Rieger's anomaly, Axenfeld anomaly,
Cone–rod dystrophy (CORD2)	*CRX*	Early-onset abnormal photoreceptor function (outer segments not developed)—autosomal dominant		Leber's amaurosis (autosomal dominant)
Cone–rod dystrophy (CORD6)	*RETGC1*	Early-onset abnormal photoreceptor function, degenerating—autosomal dominant		Leber's amaurosis autosomal recessive: severe or complete visual impairment from birth with normal fundus but extinguished ERG, pendular nystagmus

Condition	Gene			
Cone–rod dystrophy	PRPH (= RDS)	Early-onset abnormal photoreceptor function, degenerating—autosomal dominant		Later onset central retinal dystrophies, retinitis pigmentosa—autosomal dominant
Cone–rod dystrophy	RPE65	Leber's optic atrophy (recessive)		Recessive retinitis pigmentosa (later onset)
Renal Coloboma syndrome	PAX2	Optic nerve coloboma	Vesicoureteral reflux, sensorineural deafness	
Septo-optic dysplasia	HESX1	Anophthalmia	Abnormalities in the corpus callosum, the anterior and hippocampal commissures, and the septum pellucidum	Septo-optic dysplasia (one case reported)
Waardenburg syndrome type 1 and type 2	Type 1: PAX3 Type 2: MITF (15%)	Heterochromia irides	Dystopia canthorum (Waardenburg type 1), hair and skin pigmentation abnormalities, deafness, limb anomalies in severe PAX3 mutations	
Alagille syndrome	JAG1	Posterior embryotoxon	Neonatal jaundice, cholestasis, liver disease, heart disease, pulmonic valvular stenosis, peripheral pulmonary arterial stenosis, butterfly vertebrae, typical facies	

From van Heyningen V. Developmental eye disease—a genome era paradigm. Clin Genet 1998;54(4):272–82; with permission.

seem to be associated with haploinsufficiency. *CRX*, *RETGC1*, and *RPE65* have been associated with Leber congenital amaurosis, severe congenital loss of electroretinogram function, with absence of photoreceptor outer segments, but an otherwise normal fundus. This phenotype is autosomal recessive for *RETGC1* and *RPE65*, and autosomal dominant for the *CRX* gene [5].

PAX2 is a member of the paired box family which, with heterozygous loss of function, has been implicated in ocular–renal disease, and specifically contributes to optic nerve coloboma, variable severity kidney disease, and deafness. *HESX1*, another paired-type homeobox gene, has been implicated in septo-optic dysplasia of homozygous mutation origin. *PAX3*, a third paired box/homeobox protein, is associated with Waardenburg syndrome type 1. In the case of a small deletion resulting in a loss of function *JAG1* *(jagged1)*, a ligand in the *Notch* cell surface signaling pathway, has been implicated in Alagille syndrome, a multisystem disorder characterized by the ocular finding of posterior embryotoxon, or prominent Schwalbe line [5].

Many other developmental eye diseases, including some of great clinical significance or frequency, await genetic characterization. Some of these include the isolated and syndromic microphthalmias, anophthalmia, numerous colobomata, and several congenital lens and corneal diseases [5].

Summary

Congenital malformations may affect any part of the eye and ocular adnexa. Developmental defects may occur in isolation or as part of a larger systemic malformation syndrome. Congenital anomalies are of numerous origins, most commonly of developmental genetic origin. The genetic basis of congenital eye and orbit anomalies is just beginning to be characterized, and future research on the subject will undoubtedly broaden understanding of the developmental etiology, pathophysiology, and treatment of congenital ocular disease.

References

[1] Levin AV. Congenital eye anomalies. Pediatr Clin North Am 2003;50(1):55–76.
[2] Dollfus H, Verloes A. Dysmorphology and the orbital region: a practical clinical approach. Surv Ophthalmol 2004;49(6):547–61.
[3] Epstein CJ. The new dysmorphology: application of insights from basic developmental biology to the understanding of human birth defects. Proc Natl Acad Sci U S A 1995;92: 8566–73.
[4] Opitz JM. The developmental field concept in clinical genetics. J Pediatr 1982;101(5):805–9.
[5] van Heyningen V. Developmental eye disease—a genome era paradigm. Clin Genet 1998; 54(4):272–82.
[6] Bron AJ, Tripathi RC, Tripathi BJ. In: Wolff's anatomy of the eye and orbit. 8th edition. London: Chapman and Hall; 1997:620–64.

[7] Edward DP, Kaufman LM. Anatomy, development, and physiology of the visual system. Pediatr Clin North Am 2003;50(1):1–23.

[8] Cepko CL, Austin CP, Yang XY, et al. Cell fate determination in the vertebrate retina. Proc Natl Acad Sci U S A 1996;93:589–95.

[9] Amendt BA, Semina EV, Alward WL. Rieger syndrome: a clinical, molecular, and biochemical analysis. Cell Mol Life Sci 2000;57(11):1652–66.

[10] Nishimura DY, Searby CC, Alward WL, et al. A spectrum of FOXC1 mutations suggests gene dosage as a mechanism for developmental defects of the anterior chamber of the eye. Am J Hum Genet 2001;68(2):364–72.

[11] Smith RS, Zabaleta A, Kume T, et al. Haploinsufficiency of the transcription factors FOXC1 and FOXC2 results in aberrant ocular development. Hum Mol Genet 2000;9(7):1021–32.

[12] Ivanov I, Shuper A, Shohat M. Aniridia: recent achievements in paediatric practice. Eur J Pediatr 1995;154(10):795–800.

[13] Plager DA, Yang S, Neely D, et al. Complications in the first year following cataract surgery with and without IOL in infants and older children. J AAPOS 2002;6(3):133–5.

[14] Gundlach KK, Guthoff RF, Hingst VH, et al. Expansion of the socket and orbit for congenital clinical anophthalmia. Plast Reconstr Surg 2005;116(5):1214–22.

[15] Forrester MB, Merz RD. Descriptive epidemiology of anophthalmia and microphthalmia, Hawaii, 1986-2001. Birth Defects Res Part A Clin Mol Teratol 2006;76(3):187–92.

[16] Stromland K. Ocular involvement in the fetal alcohol syndrome. Surv Ophthalmol 1987; 31(4):277–84.

[17] Feingold M, Bossert WH. Normal values for selected physical parameters: an aid to syndrome delineation. Birth Defects Orig Artic Ser 1974;10(13):1–16.

[18] Farkas LG, Ross RB, Posnick JC, et al. Orbital measurements in 63 hyperteloric patients. Differences between the anthropometric and cephalometric findings. J Craniomaxillofac Surg 1989;17(6):249–54.

[19] Ward RE, Jamison PL, Farkas LG. Craniofacial variability index: a simple measure of normal and abnormal variation in the head and face. Am J Med Genet 1998;80(3):232–40.

[20] Denis D, Genitori L, Bardeot J, et al. Ocular findings in trigonocephaly. Graefe's Arch Clin Exp Ophthalmol 1994;232(12):728–33.

[21] Golden JA. Holoprosencephaly: a defect in brain patterning. J Neuropathol Exp Neurol 1998;57(11):991–9.

[22] Cohen MM, Lemire RJ. Syndromes with cephaloceles. Teratology 1982;25(2):161–72.

[23] Guion-Almeida ML, Richieri-Costa A, Saavedra D, et al. Frontonasal dysplasia: analysis of 21 cases and literature review. Int J Oral Maxillofac Surg 1996;25(2):91–7.

[24] Saavedra D, Richieri-Costa A, Guion-Almeida ML, et al. Craniofrontonasal syndrome: study of 41 patients. Am J Med Genet 1996;61(2):147–51.

[25] Mustardé J. Epicanthal folds and the problem of telecanthus. Trans Ophthalmol Soc UK 1963;83:397–411.

[26] Waardenburg PJ. A new syndrome combining developmental anomalies of the eyelids, eyebrows and nose root with pigmentary defects of the iris and head hair and with congenital deafness. Am J Hum Genet 1951;3:195–253.

[27] Read AP, Newton VE. Waardenburg syndrome. J Med Genet 1997;34(8):656–65.

[28] Snead MP, Yates JR. Clinical and molecular genetics of Stickler syndrome. J Med Genet 1999;36(5):353–9.

[29] al-Gazali LI, Farndon P, Burn J. The Schinzel-Giedion syndrome. J Med Genet 1990;27(1): 42–7.

[30] Nance MA, Berry SA. Cockayne syndrome: review of 140 cases. Am J Med Genet 1992; 42(1):68–84.

[31] Biesecker LG, Happle R, Mulliken JB. Proteus syndrome: diagnostic criteria, differential diagnosis, and patient evaluation. Am J Med Genet 1999;84(5):389–95.

[32] Price NJ, Pugh RE, Farndon PA, et al. Ablepharon macrostomia syndrome. Br J Ophthalmol 1991;75(5):317–9.

[33] Jordan DR, Anderson RL. Epicanthal folds: a deep tissue approach. Arch Ophthalmol 1989; 107(10):1532–5.

[34] Atchaneeyasakul LO, Linck LM, Connor WE, et al. Eye findings in 8 children and a spontaneously aborted fetus with RSH/Smith-Lemli-Opitz syndrome. Am J Med Genet 1998;80(5): 501–5.

[35] Lee NB, Kelly L, Sharland M. Ocular manifestations of Noonan syndrome. Eye 1992;6(3): 328–34.

[36] Clauser L, Galie M, Hassanipour A, et al. Saethre-Chotzen syndrome: review of the literature and report of a case. J Craniofac Surg 2000;11(5):480–6.

[37] Strachan T. Cornelia de Lange syndrome and the link between chromosomal function, DNA repair and developmental gene regulation. Curr Opin Genet Dev 2005;15(3): 258–64.

[38] Zlotogora J, Sagi M, Cohen T. The blepharophimosis, ptosis, and epicanthus inversus syndrome: delineation of two types. Am J Hum Genet 1983;35(5):1020–7.

[39] Ohdo S, Madokoro H, Sonada T, et al. Mental retardation associated with congenital heart disease, blepharophimosis, blepharoptosis, and hypoplastic teeth. J Med Genet 1986;23(3): 242–4.

[40] Moncla A, Philip N, Mattei JF. Blepharophimosis-mental retardation syndrome and terminal deletion of chromosome 3p. J Med Genet 1995;32(3):245–6.

[41] Yip CC, McCann JD, Goldberg RA. The role of midface lift and lateral canthal repositioning in the management of euryblepharon. Arch Ophthalmol 2004;122(7):1075–7.

[42] Niikawa N, Matsuura N, Fukushima Y, et al. Kabuki make-up syndrome: a syndrome of mental retardation, unusual facies, large and protruding ears, and postnatal growth deficiency. J Pediatr 1981;99(4):565–9.

[43] Miller MT, Deutsch TA, Cronin C, et al. Amniotic bands as a cause of ocular anomalies. Am J Ophthalmol 1987;104(3):270–9.

[44] Dixon MJ. Treacher Collins syndrome. J Med Genet 1995;32(10):806–8.

[45] Chandler KE, Kidd A, Al-Gazali L, et al. Diagnostic criteria, clinical characteristics, and natural history of Cohen syndrome. J Med Genet 2003;40(4):233–41.

[46] Weiss AH, Riscile G, Kousseff BG. Ankyloblepharon filiforme adnatum. Am J Med Genet 1992;42(3):369–73.

[47] Hay RJ, Wells RS. The syndrome of ankyloblepharon, ectodermal defects and cleft lip and palate: an autosomal dominant condition. Br J Dermatol 1976;94(3):277–89.

[48] Lacombe D. Le syndrome de Rubinstein-Taybi. Arch Pediatr 1994;1(7):681–3.

[49] Oliver GL, McFarlane DC. Congenital trichomegaly with associated pigmentary degeneration of the retina, dwarfism, and mental retardation. Arch Ophthalmol 1965;74:169–71.

[50] Moshegov CN. Ectrodactyly-ectodermal dysplasia-clefting (EEC) syndrome. Arch Ophthalmol 1996;114(10):1290–1.

[51] Mangion J, Rahman N, Mansour S, et al. A gene for lymphedema-distichiasis maps to 16q24.3. Am J Hum Genet 1999;65(2):427–32.

ELSEVIER
SAUNDERS

Otolaryngol Clin N Am
40 (2007) 141–160

OTOLARYNGOLOGIC
CLINICS
OF NORTH AMERICA

Congenital Malformations
of the Oral Cavity

Darryl T. Mueller, MD[a],*,
Vincent P. Callanan, MD, FRCS[b]

[a]*Department of Otolaryngology-Head and Neck Surgery, Temple University School
of Medicine, 3400 North Broad Street, Kresge West Building, Suite 102,
Philadelphia, PA 19140, USA*
[b]*Department of Otolaryngology-Head and Neck Surgery, Pediatric Otolaryngology,
Temple University, Temple University Children's Medical Center,
3400 North Broad Street, Kresge West Building, Suite 102,
Philadelphia, PA 19140, USA*

Congenital malformations of the oral cavity may involve the lips, jaws, hard palate, floor of mouth, and anterior two thirds of the tongue. These malformations may be the product of errors in embryogenesis or the result of intrauterine events disturbing embryonic and fetal growth [1]. This article begins with a review of the pertinent embryologic development of these structures. After reviewing the normal embryology, specific malformations are described. Recommended management follows the brief description of each malformation. An attempt is made to point out where these malformations deviate from normal development. Finally, management recommendations are based on traditional methods and recent advances described in the literature.

Embryology

Oral cavity

One can begin to see the early features of facial development by 3 weeks' gestation. At this time, the pharyngeal arches can be seen bulging out laterally from the embryo. The open ends of the arches face posteriorly and surround the upper end of the foregut and part of the primitive oral cavity or

* Corresponding author.
E-mail address: dmueller@ent.temple.edu (D.T. Mueller).

0030-6665/07/$ - see front matter © 2007 Elsevier Inc. All rights reserved.
doi:10.1016/j.otc.2006.10.007

stomodeum. The common wall of the stomodeum and foregut is known as the buccopharyngeal membrane. This membrane is found between the region of the future palatine tonsils and of the posterior third of the tongue. Normally, the buccopharyngeal membrane breaks down at approximately 4.5 weeks' gestation, establishing the connection between the oral cavity and the digestive tract [2].

Mandible and maxilla

The first pharyngeal arch, or mandibular arch, begins to grow anteriorly at 3 weeks' gestation. This arch can be subdivided into a mandibular process below and a maxillary process above. Growth centers become organized at the tips of these arches through neural crest cell migration, vascularization, and mesodermal myoblastic ingrowth. These growth centers are responsible for closing the gap between left and right paired arches [3]. The tips of the mandibular processes fuse at about 4 weeks, forming the mandible and lower lip.

Development of the upper lip and palate involves the maxillary processes and the medial nasal processes, which form at 4 weeks as the nasal pits deepen. The maxillary and medial nasal processes begin to fuse at their lower ends to form the nasal fin. This nasal fin then perforates, and connective tissue flows in to fill the groove between the right and left sides. Through cellular migration upper lip connective tissue increases and slowly fills the groove. By approximately 6 weeks, the maxillary and medial nasal processes have fused in the midline, forming the upper lip and primary palate. The nasal pits deepen until they open into the primitive oral cavity. Palatal embryology is covered in greater detail in the article by Arosarena in this issue.

Tongue

The tongue at 4 weeks has two lateral lingual swellings and one medial swelling, the tuberculum impar. These three swellings originate from the first branchial arch. A second median swelling, the copula or hypobranchial eminence, is formed by mesoderm from the second, third, and part of the fourth arch. As the lateral lingual swellings increase in size, they overgrow the tuberculum impar and merge, forming the anterior two thirds, or body, of the tongue. The posterior one third of the tongue originates from the second, third, and part of the fourth pharyngeal arch. The intrinsic tongue muscles develop from myoblasts originating in occipital somites. The body of the tongue is separated from the posterior third by a V-shaped groove, the terminal sulcus. In the midline of the terminal sulcus lies the foramen cecum, where the thyroid gland appears as an epithelial proliferation between the tuberculum impar and the copula. Later, the thyroid descends anterior to the pharyngeal gut as a bilobed diverticulum. During this migration, the thyroid remains connected to the tongue by a narrow canal, the thyroglossal duct. Normally, this duct later disappears [4].

Mandibular fusion anomalies

Median mandibular cleft

Clefts of the lower face pass through the midline of the lip and mandible (Fig. 1). Although paramedian lower lip and mandibular clefting have been reported, there are fewer than 70 cases in the literature, appearing with less frequency than the oblique facial clefts. A range of inferior clefting has been reported that extends from mild notching of the lower lip and mandibular alveolus to complete cleavage of the mandible, extending into inferior neck structures. Tongue involvement is typical although variable in expression, ranging from a bifid anterior tip with ankyloglossia to the bony cleft margins, to marked lingual hypoplasia. Inferior cervical defects (midline separation, hypoplasia, and agenesis) of the epiglottis, strap muscles, hyoid bone, thyroid cartilage, and sternum may also be present, particularly when a cutaneous cleft passes caudal to the gnathion of the chin. Median mandibular clefts result from failed coaptation of the free ends of the mandibular processes. As the incisor teeth are frequently missing along the medial mandibular margins, this suggests partial or complete failure of growth center differentiation and development rather than a simple fusion defect [3].

The lack of a consensus on the nature and timing of corrective surgery for mandibular clefts can be explained by their rarity and variability. Most authors propose correction of the soft tissue structures as soon as possible so as not to cause feeding or speech problems and mandibular bone grafting when the child is 8 to 10 years old to avoid damaging developing tooth buds. Successful management of a complete cleft of the lower lip and mandible in a one-stage procedure in the first 2 years of life has been described, however [5].

Micrognathia

Micrognathia, literally abnormal smallness of the jaws, usually refers to a small mandible. Decreased mandibular size can occur as an isolated entity

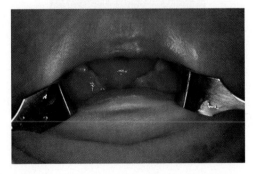

Fig. 1. Median mandibular cleft without lower lip involvement. (*Courtesy of* Glenn Isaacson, MD, Philadelphia, PA.)

or as part of a recognized syndrome. Congenital micrognathia and glossoptosis are most commonly seen in patients who have Robin sequence, but may also be associated with disorders such as Treacher Collins syndrome, Nager syndrome, and hemifacial microsomia. Infants who have Robin sequence typically have a U-shaped palatal cleft secondary to the tongue interfering with closure of the palatal processes during embryogenesis (Fig. 2). Most children born with micrognathia are asymptomatic or can be treated conservatively with prone positioning and nasopharyngeal airways. Still, up to 23% of children who have Robin sequence may have major respiratory obstruction. Tracheotomy is performed in up to 12% of patients who have severe upper airway obstruction related to micrognathia [6].

Mandell and colleagues [6] recommend mandibular distraction osteogenesis as an alternative to tracheotomy. They concluded that tracheotomy may be avoided in infants who have isolated Robin sequence and that obstructive sleep apnea can be relieved in older micrognathic children. Mandibular distraction osteogenesis is not sufficient to permit decannulation in previously tracheotomized patients who have complex congenital syndromes. Chigurupati and Myall [7] emphasize that most cases of airway obstruction attributable to isolated micrognathia can be managed with surgery. In children who have complete disease, interventions, such as tongue–lip adhesion or tracheotomy, may be preferable to mandibular distraction. Children who have craniofacial microsomia, velocardiofacial syndrome with significant pharyngeal hypotonia, Treacher Collins syndrome, or Nager syndrome may not benefit from distraction during the neonatal period because of frequent airway and temporomandibular joint anomalies.

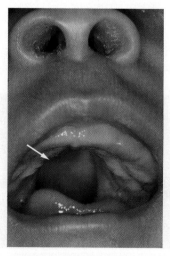

Fig. 2. Arrow points to U-shaped palatal cleft secondary to Robin sequence. (*Courtesy of* Glenn Isaacson, MD, Philadelphia, PA.)

Maxillary fusion anomalies

Cleft lip and palate

As discussed previously, fusion of the components of the upper lip and palate occurs later in embryogenesis and is more complex than that of the lower lip. Clefting anomalies of these structures are therefore more common and more varied. A comprehensive review of cleft lip and palate malformations may be found in the article by Arosarena in this issue.

Nonodontogenic (fissural) cysts

The nomenclature for cysts of the jaws and palate has changed within the past 10 to 15 years. Fissural cysts are now classified as nonodontogenic cysts. Several, including globulomaxillary, median palatal, median alveolar, and median mandibular cysts, are no longer believed to exist. Accepted nonodontogenic cysts include midpalatal cysts of infancy, nasopalatine duct cysts, and nasolabial cysts.

Midpalatal cysts of infancy, or Epstein's pearls, are keratin-filled cysts that occur in the midpalatine raphe region near the mucosal surface. They are usually seen at the junction of the hard and soft palates in the midline and not seen on the posterior soft palate (Fig. 3). The origin is believed to be epithelial inclusions that persist at the site of fusion of the opposing palatal shelves. They typically number from one to six and are just visible up to 3 mm in diameter. Cysts are noticed at birth or appear after a few days, with new ones appearing up to 2 months, but all of them disappear by 3 months. Management is by observation, because these cysts spontaneously regress. Richard and colleagues [8] caution that a double row of midline palatal cysts may be associated with an underlying submucous cleft palate.

Nasopalatine duct cysts are unilocular, often asymptomatic cysts of the anterior maxilla usually located between the roots of the central incisors.

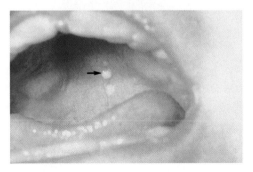

Fig. 3. Arrow points to one of three Epstein's pearls in typical midline location at the junction of the hard and soft palate.

These cysts arise from remnants of the embryonic nasopalatine duct epithelium within the nasopalatine canal. They can produce a heart-shaped radiolucency in a maxillary occlusal radiograph when the anterior nasal spine is superimposed on a central, spherical radiolucency (Fig. 4). Surgical excision of the cyst, which is lined by squamous, respiratory, or both types of epithelium, is curative [9].

The nasolabial cyst is microscopically similar to nasopalatine duct cysts but is less common and occurs in the soft tissues of the upper lip at the ala of the nose. It was considered a fusional cyst, but is now believed to arise from remnants of the nasolacrimal duct. Treatment is surgical excision [9].

Oral vestibule anomalies

Labial frenula and oral synechiae

Abnormal labial frenula may involve the upper or lower lips. In infancy, the maxillary labial frenulum typically extends over the alveolar ridge to form a raphe that reaches the palatal papilla. If this persists after the eruption of teeth it may result in a spreading of the medial incisors. Similarly, if the mandibular labial frenulum extends to the interdental papilla, its traction can lead to periodontal disease and bone loss. Each type of aberrant frenulum can be treated with surgical division when clinically significant.

Congenital oral synechiae can occur between the hard palate and floor of mouth, the tongue, or the oropharynx. These are believed to arise from persistence of the buccopharyngeal membrane that separates the mouth from the pharynx in the developing embryo [10].

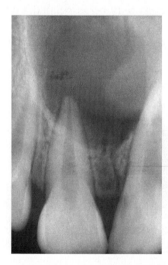

Fig. 4. Plain radiograph demonstrating central spherical radiolucency typical of nasopalatine duct cyst.

Lip pits

Congenital lip pits are rare. Three types are described, based on location: (1) commissural, (2) midline upper lip, and (3) lower lip. They occur either as an isolated defect or in association with other developmental disturbances, such as popliteal pterygium, van der Woude syndrome, oral-facial-digital syndrome, and Marres and Cremers syndromes [11]. Lip pits are depression sinuses lined by stratified squamous epithelium that communicate with minor salivary glands through their excretory ducts. Viscous saliva can be expressed from the pits when pressure is applied. Lip pits may be excised surgically to control infections or for cosmetic reasons [12].

van der Woude syndrome is an autosomal dominant condition in which lower lip pits are found in combination with cleft lip or palate. The lip pits are bilateral and symmetric paramedian depressions on the vermilion of the lower lip (Fig. 5). Recent genetic studies have shown microdeletions at chromosome bands 1q32–q41 to be the cause of van der Woude syndrome in some families. The trait may be expressed as a submucous cleft palate or the palate may be normal in affected individuals Paramedian lip pits also may be a feature of the popliteal pterygium syndrome, characterized by popliteal webbing (pterygia), cleft lip or cleft palate, genital abnormalities, and congenital bands connecting the upper and lower jaws [13].

Astomia and microstomia

Astomia results from complete union of the upper and lower lips. Microstomia refers to the rudimentary oral aperture sometimes seen in association with holoprosencephaly [14]. Congenital syndromes associated with microstomia include Hallermann-Streiff syndrome, oro-palatal dysplasia, Fine-Lubinsky syndrome, and hemifacial microsomia (Fig. 6). Perhaps the most dramatically small mouths appear in children who have Freeman-Sheldon

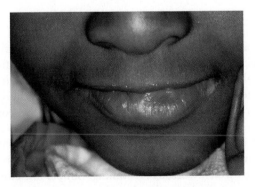

Fig. 5. Bilateral paramedian lower lip pits in a patient who has van der Woude syndrome. (*Courtesy of* Glenn Isaacson, MD, Philadelphia, PA.)

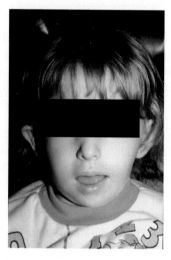

Fig. 6. Patient who has hemifacial microsomia demonstrating minimal microstomia. (*Courtesy of* Glenn Isaacson, MD, Philadelphia, PA.)

syndrome, or craniocarpotarsal dysplasia, frequently referred to as whistling baby syndrome.

Therapy for congenital microstomia is directed toward the underlying structural abnormality. The oral aperture may be widened by stair-step lengthening of the muscle in patients who have a congenitally small orbicularis oris, such as those with Freeman-Sheldon syndrome. Free flap reconstruction can interpose tissue to expand the oral opening if inadequate tissue is present. Correction of maxillary and mandibular deficiencies may correct oral asymmetry in some patients who have hemifacial microsomia. Although surgery is often required, oral expansion devices may provide enough widening to avoid invasive procedures [15].

Macrostomia

Congenital macrostomia, also known as transverse facial cleft, is a rare facial developmental anomaly. It is often associated with first or first and second branchial arch syndromes. Surgical correction involves symmetric placement of the oral commissure, reconstruction of the orbicularis oris muscle to restore labial function, reconstruction of the commissure with a normal-appearing contour, closure of the buccal defect with a minimally visible scar, and prevention of future scar contracture with lateral migration of the commissure. Z-plasty closure of the skin defect was found to yield an unacceptable scar, which worsens on smiling. Simple line closure of the skin defect gives the most aesthetically pleasing result at rest and while smiling [16].

Oral tongue anomalies

Ankyloglossia

Ankyloglossia is the result of a short, fibrous lingual frenum or a highly attached genioglossus muscle, which may be partial or complete. Incidence ranges from 0.04% to 0.1% with an equal male to female ratio. Diagnosis is made when the tongue cannot contact the hard palate and when it cannot protrude more than 1 to 2 mm past the mandibular incisors (Fig. 7A). Complete ankyloglossia is present when there is a total fusion between the tongue and floor of mouth (Fig. 7B). Diagnosis of ankyloglossia should not be made before development of the primary dentition, because the infant tongue tip is not fully developed and appears short.

Indications for surgery include presence of a speech impediment, feeding difficulty, periodontal pocketing, or psychologic problems. Correction should be delayed until the child is 4 years old because of the possibility of spontaneous elongation of the tongue as it is used in normal articulation. General anesthesia or conscious sedation is needed for younger patients. Nerve block or local infiltration is usually adequate for older patients. After identification of the submandibular duct papillae, the incision is carried posteriorly until the tip of the tongue can contact the palate and extend beyond the incisors [17].

Ankyloglossia superior is an uncommon variant in which the tongue is attached to the hard palate. If this situation occurs in conjunction with limb or maxillofacial malformations, the condition is known as ankyloglossia superior syndrome. This entity has also been associated with subglossal ankylosis, cleft palate, anencephaly, tracheoesophageal fistula, and patent foramen ovale. Surgical division under local anesthesia mobilizes the tongue [18].

Tongue fissures

Fissuring of the tongue, or lingua plicata, is believed to be an inherited trait found in 0.5% to 5% of the general population. When found in

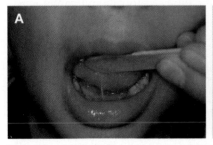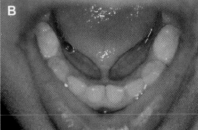

Fig. 7. (*A*) This patient who had partial ankyloglossia was unable to extend his tongue tip beyond the central mandibular incisors. (*B*) Almost complete fusion of the tongue and floor of mouth in this patient who had near total ankyloglossia. (*Courtesy of* Glenn Isaacson, MD, Philadelphia, PA.)

association with persistent and recurrent orofacial swelling and facial nerve palsy it may be part of the Melkersson-Rosenthal syndrome, a rare granulomatous disease of unknown cause. No specific therapy is required for tongue fissures alone, although brushing the tongue surface should be advised to remove any trapped food particles. Patients who have Melkersson-Rosenthal syndrome should be screened for Crohn's disease and hairy cell leukemia because of a possible association with these diseases. Therapeutic regimens for Melkersson-Rosenthal syndrome, including salazosulfapyridine, antihistamines, antibiotics, and irradiation, have met with limited success. Systemic or intralesional steroids may provide some benefit, and methotrexate has been reported to resolve symptoms dramatically. Facial nerve decompression may be indicated in cases of Melkersson-Rosenthal syndrome with recalcitrant nerve palsy [19].

Median rhomboid glossitis

Median rhomboid glossitis presents as a well-demarcated, depapillated, pink- to plum-colored patch on the dorsal surface of the tongue. This patch may be round to rhomboid in shape and ranges from 0.5 to 2.0 cm wide. Most lesions are found immediately anterior to the foramen cecum at the location of the embryologic tuberculum impar, but may present off-center or more posteriorly. Some patients describe persistent pain, irritation, or pruritus, whereas others remain asymptomatic. Cause has traditionally been considered developmental because of its consistent location at the site of the tuberculum impar. Recent investigations of its epidemiology and histopathology have suggested an infectious association, however. Candida has been recovered in a high proportion of biopsy specimens in more than one study. Also, the occurrence of median rhomboid glossitis in patients who had diabetes was significantly higher than in matched controls [20].

Treatment involves observation and follow-up for asymptomatic cases. Screening for diabetes or other immunocompromised states, in which the incidence of candidiasis is high, should be considered. Finally, symptomatic, persistent, or suspicious cases should be biopsied to rule out carcinoma.

Lingual thyroid

Ectopic thyroid tissue develops because of failed or incomplete descent of thyroid tissue during embryogenesis. The tissue can be located at any point along the normal path of descent from the foramen cecum to the low neck; however, 90% are found at the posterior tongue in the midline. Prevalence is 1 in 200,000 in the general population and 1 in 6000 patients who have thyroid disease. Lingual thyroid is seen more frequently in women and often represents the only functioning thyroid tissue. Patients may be euthyroid, hypothyroid, or hyperthyroid, and thyroid malignancies have been reported. Symptoms may present in infancy with respiratory distress or airway obstruction [21] or later in life with dysphagia, dysphonia, hemoptysis, and respiratory difficulty, including obstructive sleep apnea [22]. Patients may remain asymptomatic until the gland enlarges because of hypertrophy or malignancy.

A radionuclide thyroid scan can confirm functioning thyroid tissue in the normal location or other ectopic locations and help to differentiate ectopic thyroid from a thyroglossal duct cyst. Treatment options for symptomatic lingual thyroid may include hormone suppressive therapy, radioactive iodine ablation, or surgical excision. Thyroid supplementation must be given post-operatively if the resected lingual thyroid is the only source of endogenous thyroid hormone. In asymptomatic patients, long-term follow-up is advised.

Macroglossia

Causes of congenital enlargement of the tongue include vascular malformations (Fig. 8), hemihyperplasia, cretinism, Beckwith-Wiedemann syndrome, Down syndrome, mucopolysaccharidoses, neurofibromatosis, and multiple endocrine neoplasia, type 2B. Severity can range from mild to severe, with drooling, speech impairment, difficulty eating, stridor, and airway obstruction.

Macroglossia is a consistent manifestation of Beckwith-Wiedemann syndrome, which also may include omphalocele, visceromegaly, gigantism, neonatal hypoglycemia, and visceral tumors. Eight-five percent of these cases are sporadic and 10% to 15% have autosomal dominant inheritance with preferential maternal transmission [23].

In patients who have Beckwith-Wiedemann or hypothyroidism, the tongue shows a diffuse, smooth, generalized enlargement, whereas other forms of macroglossia usually demonstrate a multinodular appearance. Exceptional cases include lymphangiomas, in which the tongue surface is pebbly and exhibits multiple vesicle-like blebs that represent superficial dilated lymphatic channels. In Down syndrome the tongue shows a papillary,

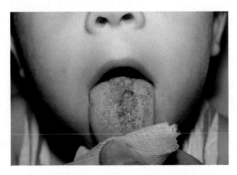

Fig. 8. Mild macroglossia secondary to lingual hemangioma. (*Courtesy of* Richard Rosenfeld, MD, Brooklyn, NY.)

fissured surface. In patients who have hemifacial hyperplasia, the enlargement is unilateral [13].

Treatment depends on severity of the condition. Surgical reduction of the tongue may be indicated in cases of congenital macroglossia, Beckwith-Wiedemann syndrome, and before or after orthodontic treatment or orthognathic surgery. Many surgical incisions have been proposed, including peripheral excisions, V-shaped wedge from the tongue tip, and an ellipse taken from the midline. Peripheral excision leaves the tongue globular and immobile, whereas V-shaped wedge shortens the tongue but does not narrow it, and midline ellipse narrows but does not shorten it. Pichler and Trauner proposed a combination of an ellipse from the midline posteriorly and a wedge from the tip performed simultaneously. This "keyhole" excision allows both narrowing and shortening of the tongue. Taste and tongue mobility are rarely affected by tongue reduction, and formal speech therapy is rarely needed after the procedure [24].

Microglossia and aglossia

Extreme microglossia is uncommon, with fewer than 50 cases described. Isolated microglossia occurs, but most cases are found in association with limb abnormalities. Gorlin classified hypoglossia–hypodactylia syndrome, one of the oromandibular-limb hypogenesis syndromes. Cause is unknown, but might include drug or alcohol exposure during gestation, gestational hyperthermia, and multifactorial or autosomal dominant inheritance with variable expression and reduced penetrance.

Airway maintenance and nutritional support are immediate concerns. Depending on symptoms, tracheotomy with nasogastric or gastrostomy tube placement may be required. With overall growth of the infant, removal of tracheotomy and feeding tubes can be accomplished. Two reports indicate that speech defects were minor regardless of tongue size, although tracheotomized patients had delay in language development. In the more severely affected individuals, speech therapy is critical for development of speech and swallowing function. Whether tissue transfer would aid in the management of these patients is yet unproven [25].

Cysts and pseudocysts

Epidermoid and dermoid cysts

Epidermoid and dermoid cysts are benign lesions, occasionally (1.6%) located within the oral cavity. These are true cysts with a wall composed of keratinized, stratified squamous epithelium and, in the case of dermoid cysts, fibrous connective tissue containing one or more skin appendages. They usually present early in life as asymptomatic masses and are treated by simple excision. If located sublingually (Fig. 9A, B), these cysts can extend into the neck as with a plunging ranula (see later discussion). In this

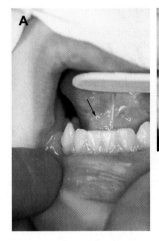
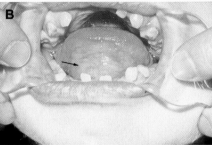

Fig. 9. (*A*) Arrow points to small sublingual dermoid cyst. (*B*) Large sublingual dermoid cyst in a patient who has Hurler syndrome.

case, surgical approach should be directed by the location of the larger component. Removal of the middle third of the hyoid in continuity with a cervical dermoid is controversial [26].

Lymphoepithelial cysts

Oral lymphoepithelial cysts developing within the lymphoid aggregates located in the floor of mouth or ventral tongue. Possible causes include:

Obstruction of lymphoid crypts
Development from salivary or mucosal epithelium trapped in lymphoid
    tissue during embryogenesis
Obstruction of the excretory ducts of the sublingual or minor salivary
    glands
Secondary immune response in associated lymphoid tissue

These are true cysts with a lining of keratinized, stratified squamous epithelium. Lymphoid tissue usually encircles the cyst, but may only involve a portion of the cyst wall. Clinically, these cysts appear white to yellow, are firm or soft to palpation, and are usually asymptomatic. Treatment is simple surgical excision [13,27].

Mucoceles and ranulas

Mucoceles are common lesions of the oral mucosa resulting from leakage of salivary mucin into the surrounding soft tissues with a granulating tissue response. Because these cysts lack a true epithelial lining, they are classified as pseudocysts. The most common location is the lower lip, where 60% are found (Fig. 10). Clinically, these are usually small, fluctuant, and

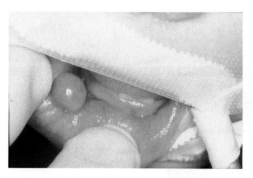

Fig. 10. Typical location of a mucocele in the vestibular portion of the paramedian lower lip.

asymptomatic mucosal swellings. Treatment consists of surgical excision with removal of the associated minor salivary gland [28].

Ranula, or "little frog," is the term given to mucoceles located within the floor of the mouth. This variety of mucocele is typically larger and caused by extravasation of mucin from the sublingual gland, or less commonly the submandibular duct or minor salivary glands in the floor of the mouth. Histology is similar to mucoceles located elsewhere in the oral cavity. Clinically, ranulas appear as blue, fluctuant swellings in the floor of the mouth lateral to the midline (Fig. 11). The term plunging ranula is given to a ranula that dissects through the mylohyoid muscle and presents within the neck (Fig. 12A). The intraoral portion of a plunging ranula may not be clinically evident, making diagnosis more difficult. Ranulas are treated by excision or marsupialization. Removal of the associated salivary gland, in this case the sublingual gland, decreases the risk for recurrence. Computed tomography may help delineate the extent of involvement preoperatively (Fig. 12B). Submental or transcervical approaches frequently are used to approach the cervical component of plunging ranulas (Fig. 12C, D) [13]. Recently transoral excision of the pseudocyst and sublingual gland or sclerotherapy with

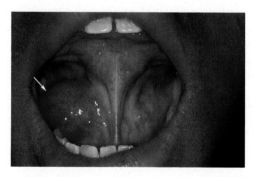

Fig. 11. Intraoral view of a large right-sided ranula. (*Courtesy of* Glenn Isaacson, MD, Philadelphia, PA.)

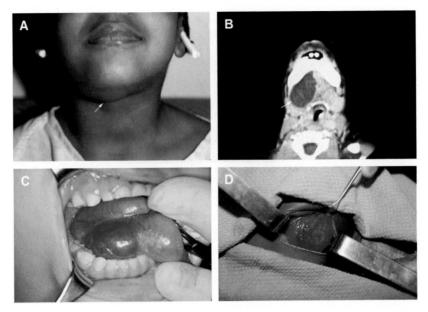

Fig. 12. (*A*) Arrow points to submental swelling suggesting ranula penetration of mylohyoid muscle. (*Courtesy of* Glenn Isaacson, MD, Philadelphia, PA.) (*B*) Noncontrast CT of same patient revealing well-circumscribed, hypodense lesion of the floor of mouth extending inferiorly to the level of the hyoid, resulting in mild airway compression. (*Courtesy of* Glenn Isaacson, MD, Philadelphia, PA.) (*C*) Ranula appearance at surgery with tongue retracted. (*Courtesy of* Richard Rosenfeld, MD, Brooklyn, NY.) (*D*) Transcervical approach was used to remove this plunging ranula. (*Courtesy of* Richard Rosenfeld, MD, Brooklyn, NY.)

OK-432 has been advocated to avoid an incision in the neck for plunging ranulas.

A rare condition that may mimic a ranula is congenital atresia of the orifice of the submandibular duct. This condition is caused by failure of hollowing of the epithelial tissue in the terminal portion of the duct during embryologic development. An imperforate duct results in accumulation of saliva, producing a cystic mass in the floor of the mouth. This lesion is a true cyst of the submandibular duct with a complete epithelial lining. Simple incision or marsupialization of these cysts has been shown to produce satisfactory results without recurrence [29].

Bohn's nodules

Bohn's nodules are inclusion cysts involving the vestibular or lingual surface of the alveolar ridge in neonates and infants. They are believed to arise from remnants of minor mucous salivary glands. These cysts cause no symptoms and may go unnoticed. They often appear between the second and fourth month of after birth and can worry parents. They may be isolated or multiple, white or translucent round papules (Fig. 13). Histologic

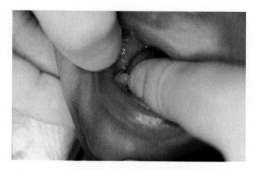

Fig. 13. Bohn's nodule of the lingual mandibular alveolar mucosa in this neonate. (*Courtesy of* Ellen Deutsch, MD, Wilmington, DE.)

examination shows true epithelial cysts containing mucous acinar cells and ducts. Treatment is not necessary, because Bohn's nodules are innocuous and disappear in a few weeks to months. Bohn's nodules should be differentiated from natal or neonatal teeth, which may be associated with several genetic disorders [30].

Benign congenital tumors

Natal teeth

Natal teeth are displaced primary tooth germs that prematurely erupt and are found at birth or within the first month of life. Mandibular central incisors are most frequently involved, followed by the maxillary incisors. An autosomal dominant pattern of inheritance may be seen. Natal teeth are associated with more than 20 syndromes, including chondroectodermal dysplasia, Noonan syndrome, pachyonychia congenita (an autosomal dominant disorder of keratinization), oculomandibulodyscephaly, and Turner syndrome.

Treatments include observation, smoothing of the incisal edge, or immediate extraction. Smoothing of the incisal edge decreases discomfort during breast feeding and prevents Riga-Fede disease, an ulceration in the floor of the mouth. Natal teeth are removed when they are excessively mobile to prevent the potential risk for aspiration. Left alone, a natal tooth becomes less mobile with development of its root [31].

Epulis

Epulis, or congenital gingival granular cell tumor, is a rare benign soft tissue tumor that appears exclusively in newborns. Females are affected more often than males (8:1 to 10:1). These typically present at birth as a pedunculated mass on the premaxillary or mandibular alveolar mucosa with solitary or multiple nodules (Fig. 14) [32]. A large epulis can interfere

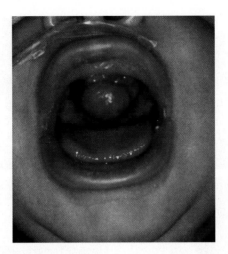

Fig. 14. Epulis located on premaxillary alveolar mucosa in a newborn. (*Courtesy of* Ellen Deutsch, MD, Wilmington, DE.)

with breathing and feeding. Reported size ranges from a few millimeters to 8 cm.

Histologically, these benign tumors are composed of diffuse sheets and clusters of polygonal cells containing round, small nuclei with abundant, coarsely granular cytoplasm. A fine vascular network between granular cells accounts for their tendency to bleed. Congenital granular cell tumors are distinguished from the more common granular cell tumors by lack of pseudoepitheliomatous hyperplasia, absence of S-100 protein expression, and positive reaction to CEA and HLA-DR antigen.

Treatment depends on tumor size and presence of any obstructive symptoms. Small, asymptomatic lesions may be observed until spontaneous regression occurs. Larger lesions interfering with feeding or breathing should be surgically excised under local or general anesthesia. If a potentially obstructing lesion is identified on prenatal ultrasound, a multidisciplinary team can be assembled to ensure airway patency at birth and effect a rapid, simple removal of the tumor by ex utero intrapartum treatment (EXIT). EXIT allows maintenance of adequate uteroplacental blood flow for up to 1 hour, giving ample time for surgical removal [33].

Heterotopia or choristoma

Heterotopia is synonymous with choristoma. These terms refer to the displacement of normal tissue or organs into an abnormal location within the body. Heterotopic tissue in the oral cavity is a rare finding, but has been described in several case reports. Various tissue types have been found, including gastric, intestinal, colonic, respiratory, neuroglial tissues, cartilage, and bone.

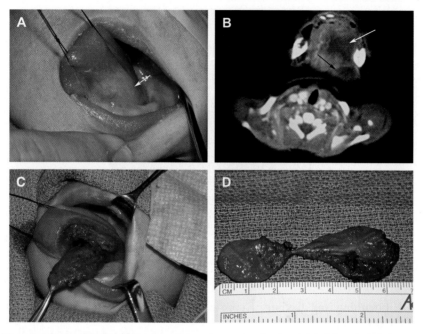

Fig. 15. (*A*) Arrow indicates heterotopic gastric mucosa–lined cyst involving the left floor of mouth and sublingual region of this 1-day-old infant. (*B*) Contrast-enhanced axial CT demonstrates a hypodense, bilobed lesion of the left floor of mouth. Open arrow points to anterior lobe. Solid arrow points to posterior lobe. (*C*) Preoperative knowledge of bilobed quality of the cyst led to further dissection at this point. (*D*) Specimen measured 6 cm in length and was bilobed as demonstrated in preoperative CT.

Heterotopic gastric tissue can be found in a gastric or enteric duplication cyst. The cause of gastric heterotopia is still unknown. The most commonly held hypothesis is misplacement or sequestration of endoderm from the gastric anlage in the developing tongue or floor of mouth around the fourth week of gestation. Among enteric duplications, gastric heterotopias are the most common [34].

These aberrant rests of tissue may present as an asymptomatic cyst or mass (Fig. 15A, B), or may cause feeding difficulties or airway obstruction. Treatment is usually simple surgical excision (Fig. 15C, D) [35].

References

[1] Jones KL. Morphogenesis and dysmorphogenesis. In: Jones KL, editor. Smith's recognizable patterns of human malformation. 5th edition. Philadelphia: WB Saunders; 1997. p. 695–705.
[2] Isselhard B. Development of orofacial complex. In: Kuhn S, Macciocca K, editors. Anatomy of orofacial structures. 7th edition. St. Louis (MO): Mosby Inc.; 2003. p. 248–51.

[3] Eppley BL, van Aalst JA, Robey A, et al. The spectrum of orofacial clefting. Plast Reconstr Surg 2005;115(7):101–14.

[4] Sadler TW. Head and neck. In: Sun B, editor. Langman's medical embryology. 9th edition. Philadelphia: Lippincott Williams & Wilkins; 2004. p. 382–90.

[5] Almeida LE, Ulbrich L, Togni F. Mandible cleft: report of a case and review of the literature. J Oral Maxillofac Surg 2002;60(6):681–4.

[6] Mandell DL, Yellon RF, Bradley JP, et al. Mandibular distraction for micrognathia and severe upper airway obstruction. Arch Otolaryngol Head Neck Surg 2004;130(3): 344–8.

[7] Chigurupati R, Myall R. Airway management in babies with micrognathia: the case against early distraction. J Oral Maxillofac Surg 2005;63(8):1209–15.

[8] Richard BM, Qiu CX, Ferguson MWJ. Neonatal palatal cysts and their morphology in cleft lip and palate. Br J Plast Surg 2000;53(7):555–8.

[9] Daley TD, Wysocki GP. New developments in selected cysts of the jaws. J Can Dent Assoc 1997;63(7):526–32.

[10] Gartlan MG, Davies J, Smith RJH. Congenital oral synechiae. Ann Otol Rhinol Laryngol 1993;102(3 Pt 1):186–97.

[11] Rizos M, Spyropoulos MN. Van der Woude syndrome: a review. Cardinal signs, epidemiology, associated features, differential diagnosis, expressivity, genetic counseling and treatment. Eur J Orthod 2004;26(1):17–24.

[12] Zarandy MM, Givehchi G, Mohammadi M. A familial occurrence of lip anomaly. Am J Otolaryngol 2005;26(2):132–4.

[13] Neville BW, Damm DD, Allen CM, et al. Developmental defects of the oral and maxillofacial region. In: Neville BW, Damm DD, Allen CM, et al, editors. Oral & maxillofacial pathology. 2nd edition. Philadelphia: WB Saunders; 2002. p. 1–73.

[14] Chervenak FA, Isaacson G, Hobbins JC, et al. Diagnosis and management of fetal holoprosencephaly. Obstet Gynecol 1985;66(3):322–6.

[15] Ferreira LM, Minami E, Andrews JM. Freeman-Sheldon syndrome: surgical correction of microstomia. Br J Plast Surg 1994;47(3):201–2.

[16] Schwarz R, Sharma D. Straight line closure of congenital macrostomia. Indian Journal of Plastic Surgery 2004;37(2):121–3.

[17] Warden PJ. Ankyloglossia: a review of the literature. Gen Dent 1991;39(4):252–3.

[18] Kalu PU, Moss ALH. An unusual case of ankyloglossia superior. Br J Plast Surg 2004;57(6): 579–81.

[19] Winnie R, DeLuke DM. Melkersson-Rosenthal syndrome review of literature and case report. Int J Oral Maxillofac Surg 1992;21(2):115–7.

[20] Carter LC. Median rhomboid glossitis: review of a puzzling entity. Compend Contin Educ Dent 1990;11(7):446–50.

[21] Chanin LR, Greenberg LM. Pediatric upper airway obstruction due to ectopic thyroid: classification and case reports. Laryngoscope 1988;98(4):422–7.

[22] Barnes TW, Olsen KD, Morgenthaler TI. Obstructive lingual thyroid causing sleep apnea: a case report and review of the literature. Sleep Med 2004;5(6):605–7.

[23] Cohen MM. Beckwith-Wiedemann syndrome: historical, clinicopathological, and etiopathogenetic perspectives. Pediatr Dev Pathol 2005;8(3):287–304.

[24] Wang J, Goodger NM, Pogrel MA. The role of tongue reduction. Oral Surg Oral Med Oral Pathol Oral Radiol Endod 2003;95(3):269–73.

[25] Thorp MA, de Waal PJ, Prescott CAJ. Extreme microglossia. Int J Pediatr Otorhinolaryngol 2003;67(5):473–7.

[26] Bitar MA, Kumar S. Plunging congenital epidermoid cyst of the oral cavity. Eur Arch Otorhinolaryngol 2003;260(4):223–5.

[27] Epivatianos A, Zaraboukas T, Antoniades D. Coexistence of lymphoepithelial and epidermoid cysts on the floor of the mouth: report of a case. Oral Dis 2005;11(5): 330–3.

[28] Andiran N, Sarikayalar F, Unal OF, et al. Mucocele of the anterior lingual salivary glands: from extravasation to an alarming mass with a benign course. Int J Pediatr Otorhinolaryngol 2001;61(2):143–7.

[29] Amin MA, Bailey BMW. Congenital atresia of the orifice of the submandibular duct: a report of 2 cases and review. Br J Oral Maxillofac Surg 2001;39(6):480–2.

[30] Cambiaghi S, Gelmetti C. Bohn's nodules. Int J Dermatol 2005;44(9):753–4.

[31] Hayes PA. Hamartomas, eruption cyst, natal tooth and Epstein pearls in a newborn. ASDC J Dent Child 2000;67(5):365–8.

[32] Merrett SJ, Crawford PJM. Congenital epulis of the newborn: a case report. Int J Paediatr Dent 2003;13(2):127–9.

[33] Kumar P, Kim HHS, Zahtz GD, et al. Obstructive congenital epulis: prenatal diagnosis and perinatal management. Laryngoscope 2002;112(11):1935–9.

[34] Wetmore RF, Bartlett SP, Papsin B, et al. Heterotopic gastric mucosa of the oral cavity: a rare entity. Int J Pediatr Otorhinolaryngol 2002;66(2):139–42.

[35] Marina MB, Zurin AR, Muhaizan WM, et al. Heterotopic neuroglial tissue presenting as oral cavity mass with intracranial extension. Int J Pediatr Otorhinolaryngol 2005;69(11): 1587–90.

ELSEVIER
SAUNDERS

Otolaryngol Clin N Am
40 (2007) 161–176

OTOLARYNGOLOGIC
CLINICS
OF NORTH AMERICA

Congenital Cervical Cysts, Sinuses and Fistulae

Stephanie P. Acierno, MD, MPH, John H.T. Waldhausen, MD*

Department of Surgery, Children's Hospital and Regional Medical Center, University of Washington School of Medicine, G0035, 4800 Sand Point Way, NE, Seattle, WA 98105, USA

Congenital cervical cysts, sinuses, and fistulae must be considered in the diagnosis of head and neck masses in children and adults. These include, in descending order of frequency, thyroglossal duct cysts, branchial cleft anomalies, dermoid cysts, and median cervical clefts. A thorough understanding of the embryology and anatomy of each of these lesions is necessary to provide accurate preoperative diagnosis and appropriate surgical therapy, which are essential to prevent recurrence. The following sections review each lesion, its embryology, anatomy, common presentation, evaluation, and the key points in surgical management.

Thyroglossal duct anomalies

Thyroglossal duct anomalies are the second most common pediatric neck mass, behind adenopathy in frequency [1]. Thyroglossal duct remnants occur in approximately 7% of the population, although only a minority of these is ever symptomatic [1].

Embryology

The thyroid gland forms from a diverticulum (median thyroid anlage) located between the anterior and posterior muscle complexes of the tongue at week 3 of gestation. As the embryo grows, the diverticulum is displaced caudally into the neck and fuses with components from the fourth and fifth

---

* Corresponding author.
E-mail address: john.waldhausen@seattlechildrens.org (J.H.T. Waldhausen).

0030-6665/07/$ - see front matter © 2007 Elsevier Inc. All rights reserved.
doi:10.1016/j.otc.2006.10.009

branchial pouches (lateral thyroid anlagen). The descent continues anterior to or through the hyoid bone with the median anlage elongating into the thyroglossal duct (Fig. 1) [2]. By weeks 5 to 8 of gestation, the thyroglossal duct obliterates, leaving a proximal remnant, the foramen cecum, at the base of the tongue and a distal remnant, the pyramidal lobe of the thyroid [1,2]. If the duct fails to obliterate before the formation of the mesodermal anlage of the hyoid bone, it persists as a cyst [2].

Clinical presentation and diagnosis

Two thirds of thyroglossal duct anomalies are diagnosed within the first 3 decades of life, with more than half being identified before age 10 years [1]. The most common presentation is that of a painless cystic neck mass near the hyoid bone in the midline (Figs. 2 and 3) [2]. Although they are most commonly found immediately adjacent to the hyoid (66%), they can also be located between the tongue and hyoid, between the hyoid and pyramidal lobe, within the tongue, or within the thyroid [2,3]. The mass usually moves with swallowing or protrusion of the tongue. Approximately one third present with a concurrent or prior infection, which is the more common presentation in adults [2,4]. One fourth of patients present with a draining sinus that results from spontaneous drainage or surgical drainage of an abscess [2]. This drainage can result in a foul taste in the mouth if the spontaneous drainage occurred by way of the foramen cecum. These lesions also fluctuate in size. Other rare presentations can be severe respiratory distress or sudden infant death syndrome from lesions at the base of the tongue, a lateral cystic neck mass, an anterior tongue fistula, or coexistence with branchial anomalies [2].

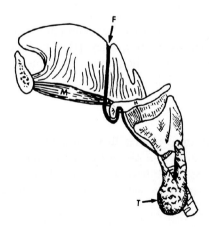

Fig. 1. The course of the thyroglossal duct extending from the foramen cecum (F) to the thyroid (T). (*From* Som PM, Smoker WRK, Curtin HD, et al. Congenital lesions in head and neck imaging. In: Som PM, Curtin HD, editors. Head and neck surgery. St. Louis: Mosby; 2003. p. 121–5; with permission.)

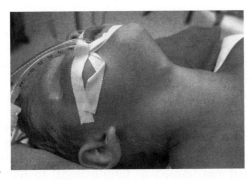

Fig. 2. Thyroglossal duct cyst, uncomplicated. (*From* Foley DS, Fallat ME. Thyroglossal duct and other congenital midline cervical anomalies. Semin Pediatr Surg 2006;15: 70–5; with permission.)

The preoperative evaluation for a patient who has a suspected thyroglossal duct cyst includes a complete history and physical examination, preoperative ultrasound, and a screening thyroid stimulating hormone (TSH) level. Patients who have history, examination findings, or elevated TSH levels suggesting hypothyroidism or a solid mass should undergo scintiscanning to rule out a median ectopic thyroid [2]. When median ectopic thyroid is present, all of the patient's functional thyroid tissue can be located within the cyst, and its removal would render the patient permanently dependent on thyroid replacement. The management of median ectopic thyroid is controversial. Some investigators believe these patients can be treated with exogenous thyroid hormone to suppress the gland, whereas others advocate for resection for reasons that are discussed later [2]. Although median ectopic thyroid only occurs in 1% to 2% of thyroglossal duct cysts, some authors advocate for scintiscans in all patients [5].

Treatment

Elective surgical excision is the treatment of choice for uncomplicated thyroglossal duct cysts to prevent infection of the cyst. The Sistrunk

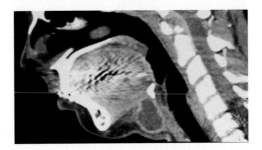

Fig. 3. Sagittal CT reconstruction of a thyroglossal duct cyst demonstrating the close relationship to the hyoid bone. (*Courtesy of* Glenn Isaacson, MD, Philadelphia, PA.)

procedure is performed, rather than simple excision, to reduce recurrence risk [2]. With the patient in supine position and the neck extended, a transverse incision is made over the mass. The dissection is carried down to the cyst, then caudally to identify the tract to the pyramidal lobe. If present, it is excised en bloc with the cyst. The surgeon then dissects cranially toward the hyoid bone and a block of tissue around the proximal tract is also excised. The central portion of the hyoid bone is also excised and the tract is further dissected with a core of tissue from the muscle at the base of the tongue to the foramen cecum (Fig. 4) [2]. After confirming adequate proximal dissection by pressure on the base of the tongue from the mouth, the tract is ligated and transected. Intrathyroidal thyroglossal duct cysts should also undergo a Sistrunk procedure if there is a transhyoidal fistulous tract, but can be treated with hemi-thyroidectomy if no tract can be identified [3].

Infected cysts or sinuses are first managed by relieving the infection. The cysts are usually infected by way of the mouth, thus the most common organisms are *Haemophilus influenza*, *Staphylococcus aureus*, and *Staphylococcus epidermidis* [2]. Antibiotics directed toward those organisms should be started. Needle aspiration may allow for decompression and identification of the organism. Formal incision and drainage should be avoided, if possible, to prevent seeding of ductal cells outside the cyst, which increases recurrence [2]. If incision and drainage is necessary, the incision should be placed so it can be completely excised with an ellipse at the time of definitive resection. Once the infection clears and the incision heals, the patient may undergo an elective Sistrunk procedure [2].

If a solid mass is encountered during excision of a suspected thyroglossal duct cyst, it should be sent for frozen section to rule out a median ectopic thyroid. If the biopsy returns as normal thyroid tissue and the patient has functional thyroid tissue in the normal location, it should be excised by

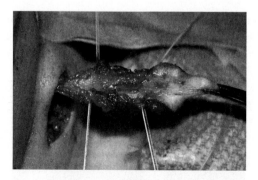

Fig. 4. Sistrunk procedure resection of a thyroglossal duct cyst; note that the specimen includes the cyst, hyoid bone, and proximal tract en bloc. (*From* Foley DS, Fallat ME. Thyroglossal duct and other congenital midline cervical anomalies. Semin Pediatr Surg 2006;15:70–5; with permission.)

the Sistrunk procedure [2]. If the mass is possibly the patient's only functional thyroid tissue, the management becomes controversial. One option involves leaving the ectopic thyroid, either in situ or repositioning it laterally below the strap muscles or into the rectus abdominus or quadriceps muscles. This option aims to not render the patient permanently hypothyroid; however, most patients still require long-term thyroid hormone therapy to treat hypothyroidism or control the size of the ectopic thyroid tissue for cosmetic or functional reasons. This need for long-term therapy and the possibility of malignant degeneration have led some to recommend excision of the median ectopic thyroid regardless of the presence of additional thyroid tissue [2].

Thyroglossal duct cysts are lined with ductal epithelium or contain solid thyroid tissue. Less than 1.0% have malignant tissue, usually well-differentiated thyroid carcinoma. This malignancy occurs more often in adults, but has been reported in children as young as 6 years old [6]. It is usually identified incidentally at the time of surgery for a suspected thyroglossal duct cyst. Papillary carcinoma is seen most often, although all types of thyroid carcinoma except medullary carcinoma have been reported [2,4]. If there is no evidence of capsular invasion or distant or regional metastasis, the Sistrunk procedure has been associated with a 95% cure rate, although careful follow-up is necessary [2]. Other investigators recommend completion thyroidectomy regardless of capsular invasion citing the benefits of full pathologic examination of the gland, facilitation of radioactive iodine ablation, and increased sensitivity of radioisotope screening for recurrence [1]. If capsular invasion is present, completion thyroidectomy, nodal dissection, and radioiodine ablation should be pursued as indicated by type and stage of disease [2].

Recurrence of thyroglossal duct cyst after complete excision using the Sistrunk procedure is reported to be 2.6% to 5% [1,4]. Several factors have been identified predisposing patients to increased risk for recurrence. Failure to completely excise the cyst (especially simple excision alone) can result in recurrence rates of 38% to 70% [1,4]. In children less than 2 years old, intraoperative cyst rupture and presence of a cutaneous component increases the risk for recurrence. Preoperative or concurrent infection of the cyst has been historically reported as a risk factor because of the increased difficulty of complete resection, although a recent review found that postoperative infections rather than preoperative infections were associated with increased recurrence [2,7]. Recurrent thyroglossal cyst excision has a higher risk for recurrence (20%–35%) and requires a wider en bloc resection [2].

Branchial cleft anomalies

Branchial anomalies compose approximately 30% of congenital neck masses and can present as cysts, sinuses, or fistulae [1,8]. They are equally common in males and females and usually present in childhood or early adulthood.

Embryology

By the end of the fourth week of gestation, there are four well-defined pairs of arches and two rudimentary arches. These are lined externally by ectoderm, internally by endoderm, with mesoderm in between. The mesoderm contains the dominant artery, nerve, cartilage rod, and muscle for each arch. Each arch is separated by clefts externally and pouches internally. In fish these structures form gills, but in humans the clefts and pouches are gradually obliterated by mesenchyme to form the mature head and neck structures (Fig. 5) [8]. Branchial anomalies result from incomplete obliteration of the clefts and pouches.

Each arch transforms throughout gestation into a defined anatomic pattern. Knowledge of this pattern of transformation and its relationship to normal structures in the neck is essential in the diagnosis and treatment of these anomalies. Branchial anomalies are classified by the cleft or pouch of origin and this is determined by the internal opening of the sinus and its relationship to nerves, arteries, and muscles. A thorough understanding of these relationships is needed to prevent injury to surrounding structures and ensure complete resection [8]. The essential embryology and anatomy is described for each cleft in later discussion.

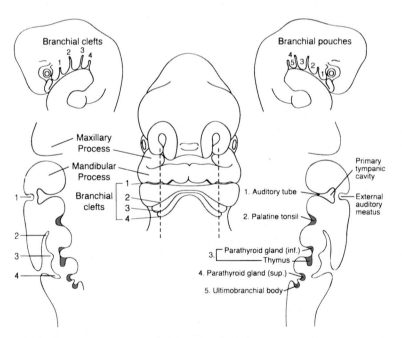

Fig. 5. Branchial embryology at the fifth week of gestation. Sagittal sections demonstrate the anatomic relationship of the external clefts and internal pouches and the derivation of important head and neck structures. (*From* Waldhausen JHT. Branchial cleft and arch anomalies in children. Semin Pediatr Surg 2006;15:64–9; with permission.)

Pathology

Branchial anomalies can be lined with either respiratory or squamous epithelium. Cysts are often lined by squamous epithelium, whereas sinuses and fistulae are more likely to be lined with ciliated, columnar epithelium [8]. Lymphoid tissue, sebaceous glands, salivary tissue, or cholesterol crystals in mucoid fluid can also be seen. Squamous cell cancer can be found within branchial lesions in adults, although it is rare. It is difficult to distinguish between a primary lesion arising from within an anomaly and a metastatic lesion from an occult primary [1].

Diagnosis

Branchial anomalies can present as cysts, sinuses, or fistulae. Cysts are remnants of the cervical sinus without an external opening. Sinuses are the persistence of the cervical sinus with its external opening, whereas a fistula also involves persistence of the branchial groove with breakdown of the branchial membrane resulting in a pharyngocutaneous fistula [1]. The specific presentation for each cleft is described in later discussion.

The evaluation of these lesions begins with a complete history and physical, which may include upper airway endoscopy to locate the pharyngeal opening. The pyriform sinus and the tonsillar fossa should be carefully examined. In adults, fine needle aspiration should be performed to rule out metastatic carcinoma or clarify the diagnosis [8]. This clarification is not necessary in children and incisional biopsy should not be performed because this makes the resection more difficult. Ultrasound, CT, and MRI can be used to help define the lesion and its course, but CT is the current study of choice. Current tomography is able to demonstrate the fistula in up to 64% of cases [9]. Barium esophagram can also be helpful with a 50% to 80% sensitivity for third and fourth branchial fistulae [10].

Treatment

The definitive treatment of all branchial anomalies is complete surgical excision. Unresected cysts and sinuses have a high risk for infection and incomplete resection results in high rates of recurrence [8]. Timing of resection is controversial with some advocating for early resection to prevent infection whereas others support waiting until age 2 to 3 years [8,11,12]. Twenty percent of lesions have been infected at least once before the time of surgery [11]. As with thyroglossal duct cysts, acute infections should first be treated with antibiotics, needle aspiration, and, if necessary, incision and drainage, followed by complete resection after resolution of the infection. Specific considerations for the resection of each type of anomaly are discussed later.

First cleft anomalies

First branchial cleft anomalies account for only 1% of branchial cleft malformations [8]. The first arch, or mandibular arch, forms the mandible, part of the maxillary process of the upper jaw, and portions of the inner ear. The first cleft and pouch form the external auditory canal, eustachian tube, middle ear cavity, and mastoid air cells. First cleft anomalies may involve either the external auditory canal or, occasionally, the middle ear [8]. First cleft anomalies course close to the parotid gland, especially the superficial lobe, traveling above, between, or below the facial nerve branches. First cleft anomalies are classified as Type I or Type II (Figs. 6 and 7). Type I lesions are duplications of the membranous external auditory canal, are composed of ectoderm only, course lateral to the facial nerve, and present as swellings near the ear. Type II lesions have ectoderm and mesoderm, can contain cartilage, pass medial to the facial nerve, and present as preauricular, infra-auricular, or postauricular swellings inferior to the angle of the mandible or anterior to the sternocleidomastoid muscle [1,8].

First cleft anomalies can present as cysts, sinuses or fistulae located between the external auditory canal and the submandibular area. They are more common in females than males and are often misdiagnosed leading to a delay in excision [13,14]. Ten percent have an asymptomatic membranous attachment from the floor of the external auditory canal to the

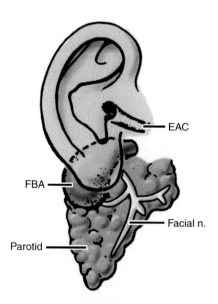

Fig. 6. Type I first branchial cleft anomaly. Note that the cyst (FBA) is located within the parotid gland and does not connect to the external auditory canal (EAC). (*From* Mukherji SK, Fatterpekar G, Castillo M, et al. Imaging of congenital anomalies of the branchial apparatus. Neuroimaging Clin N Am 2000;10:75–93; with permission.)

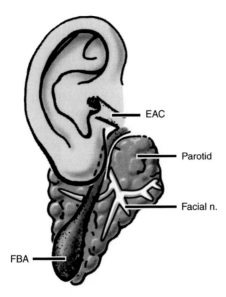

Fig. 7. Type II first branchial cleft anomaly. Note that the cyst (FBA) communicates with the external auditory canal (EAC) and extends into the deep lobe of the parotid gland. (*From* Mukherji SK, Fatterpekar G, Castillo M, et al. Imaging of congenital anomalies of the branchial apparatus. Neuroimaging Clin N Am 2000;10:75–93; with permission.)

tympanic membrane [8,13]. Presentations vary, but include cervical, parotid, or auricular signs. Cervical signs consist of drainage from a pit-like depression at the angle of the mandible, which can be purulent if infected. Parotid involvement is likely if there is rapid enlargement because of inflammation. Auricular signs include swelling or otorrhea.

The surgical resection of first arch anomalies often requires at least partial facial nerve dissection and superficial parotidectomy. It is also necessary to excise any involved skin or cartilage of the external auditory canal. If the tract extends medial to the tympanic membrane, it may be necessary to transect the tract and remove the medial portion during a second procedure. Compared with tracts that go to the external auditory canal, tracts going to the middle ear tend to lie deep to the facial nerve [9]; however, tracts can split around the nerve [13]. Recurrence is common, with the average number of procedures required to achieve complete resection being 2.4 per patient [15]. Each repeat surgery has an increased risk for injury to the facial nerve because of previous scarring, indicating the importance of complete resection at the first attempt when possible [8].

Second cleft anomalies

Second branchial cleft anomalies are the most common, representing 95% of all brachial cleft malformations. The second arch, or hyoid arch, forms the hyoid bone and adjacent areas of the neck. The second pouch gives rise to the tonsillar and supratonsillar fossae. Second cleft anomalies thus enter the supratonsillar fossa [8]. These anomalies pass close to the glossopharyngeal and hypoglossal nerves on their course to the fossa. Second arch anomalies are classified into four types as demonstrated in Fig. 8. Type I lesions lie anterior to the sternocleidomastoid muscle (SCM) and do not contact the carotid sheath. Type II lesions are the most common and pass deep to the SCM and either anterior or posterior to the carotid sheath. Type III lesions pass between the internal and external carotid arteries and are adjacent to the pharynx. Type IV lesions lie medial to the carotid sheath close to the pharynx adjacent to the tonsillar fossa.

Second brachial cleft anomalies present as a fistula or cyst in the lower, anterolateral neck. Cysts are most commonly diagnosed in adults during the third and fifth decades as a nontender mass that can acutely increase in size after an upper respiratory infection. The enlargement can lead to

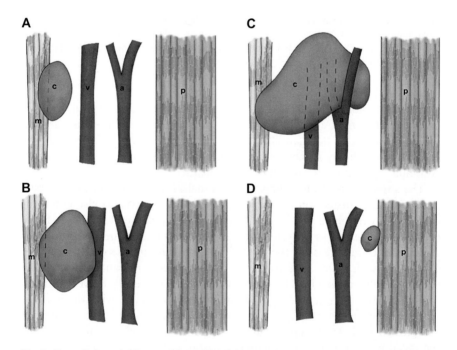

Fig. 8. Types I through IV second branchial cleft anomalies. (*A*) Type I: the cyst (C) is superficial to the anterior border of the sternocleidomastoid muscle (M). (*B*) Type II: the cyst is adjacent to the carotid sheath. (*C*) Type III: the cyst passes between the internal and external carotid arteries and extends to the lateral wall of the pharynx (P). (*D*) Type IV: the cyst is deep to the carotid sheath abutting the pharynx. (*From* Mukherji SK, Fatterpekar G, Castillo M, et al. Imaging of congenital anomalies of the branchial apparatus. Neuroimaging Clin N Am 2000;10:75–93; with permission.)

respiratory compromise, torticollis, or dysphagia. Fistulae, however, are usually diagnosed in infancy or childhood and present as chronic drainage from an opening along the anterior border of the SCM in the lower third of the neck [1,8].

Surgical resection of second cleft anomalies can be approached by way of a transverse cervical incision placed within a natural skin fold. Cysts can be located either superficially or deep to the cervical fascia. A careful exploration for an associated fistula tract must be performed with a complete excision of the entire tract if one is found. Fistula excision can be facilitated by cannulating the tract with a 2-0 or 3-0 monofilament suture or probe. The tract can also be injected with methylene blue; however this may stain the surrounding tissues making dissection difficult [8]. As the tract is followed, the skin incision may have to be extended to allow adequate exposure, although step-ladder incisions may provide improved visualization of the tract near the pharynx. The spinal accessory, hypoglossal, and vagus nerves must be protected from injury during the dissection. A finger or bougie in the oropharynx can help identify the opening in the tonsillar fossa. The thin tract must be carefully ligated and divided at its entry into the fossa. If the excision is complete, no drain is needed.

Third and fourth cleft anomalies

Third and fourth branchial anomalies are rare. The third and fourth pouches form the pharynx below the hyoid bone, thus these sinuses and fistulae enter into the pyriform sinus. Third and fourth branchial anomalies normally contain thymic tissue as do cysts and sinuses that result from thymic or parathyroid rests, but only branchial anomalies have the connection to the pyriform sinus. Third arch anomalies present as cystic structures located at the lower, anterior border of the SCM, at the level of the superior pole of the thyroid [1,8]. They pass deep to the internal carotid artery and the glossopharyngeal nerve, entering the thyroid membrane above the internal branch of the superior laryngeal nerve, then entering the pyriform sinus of the pharynx (Fig. 9). Third arch cysts can cause hypoglossal nerve palsy if infected. The course of fourth arch anomalies depends on the side (Fig. 10). On the right, the lesion loops around the subclavian artery, passes deep to the internal carotid artery, ascending to the level of the hypoglossal nerve, then descends along the anterior border of the SCM to enter the pharynx at the pyriform apex or cervical esophagus. On the left, the tract descends into the mediastinum, looping around the aortic arch, medial to the ligamentum arteriosus, then ascends in a similar course to the right side. Fourth arch lesions present as lateral cysts in the lower third of the neck [1,8]. Both third and fourth cleft lesions can present at any age. Either can also present with tracheal compression and airway compromise in the neonate because of rapid enlargement in size. Third and fourth brachial cleft cysts can also present as cold nodules in the thyroid leading to confusion with thyroglossal

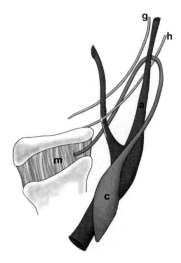

Fig. 9. Third branchial cleft anomaly. The cyst (C) is posterior to the sternocleidomastoid muscle, and the tract ascends posterior to the internal carotid artery. It then passes medially to pass between the hypoglossal (H) and glossopharyngeal (G) nerves. It pierces the thyroid membrane to enter the pyriform sinus. (*From* Mukherji SK, Fatterpekar G, Castillo M, et al. Imaging of congenital anomalies of the branchial apparatus. Neuroimaging Clin N Am 2000;10:75–93; with permission.)

duct cysts. Other possible presentations include recurrent upper respiratory tract infections, neck or thyroid pain, or thyroid abscess.

Surgical therapy of third and fourth arch anomalies is similar to that of second arch anomalies, with the following exceptions. Endoscopy should be used to identify the pyriform sinus entry point. This identification can allow cannulation or injection of the tract to aid with dissection. There are some reports of chemical cauterization of these tracts; however, there are no long-term results for this approach [16]. Fourth arch anomaly resections require ipsilateral hemithyroidectomy to completely excise the tract and possible partial resection of the thyroid cartilage to provide adequate exposure of the pyriform sinus [17].

Branchiootorenal syndrome

Branchiootorenal syndrome (BOR) or Melnick-Fraser syndrome is an autosomal dominant disorder with coinheritance of branchial arch anomalies. It occurs in approximately 2% of profoundly deaf students, with an estimated 1:40,000 to 1:700,000 prevalence [18]. It has been mapped to chromosome 8q 13.3, the human homolog of the *Drosophila* eyes absent gene that has roles in cochlear and vestibular development and renal morphogenesis [18]. The typical phenotype consists of cup-shaped pinnae; preauricular pits; branchial fistulae; conductive, sensorineural, or mixed

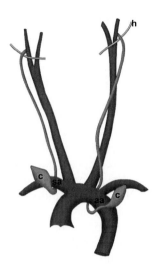

Fig. 10. Fourth branchial cleft anomaly. The cysts (C) are located anterior to the aortic arch on either side. The tract hooks either the subclavian artery or the aortic arch, depending on the side, and ascends to loop over the hypoglossal nerve (H). (*From* Mukherji SK, Fatterpekar G, Castillo M, et al. Imaging of congenital anomalies of the branchial apparatus. Neuroimaging Clin N Am 2000;10:75–93; with permission.)

hearing impairment; and renal anomalies ranging from mild hypoplasia to complete absence. Other findings may include preauricular tags, lacrimal duct stenosis, a constricted palate, a deep overbite, and a long, narrow face. Hearing loss and preauricular pits are most common, with branchial cleft fistulae occurring in approximately 50% of individuals [18].

Dermoid cysts and teratomas

Dermoid cysts result from entrapment of epithelial elements along embryonic lines of fusion (median and paramedian) and contain ectodermal and endodermal elements [1]. Dermoids are lined by epithelium but contain epithelial appendages, such as hair, hair follicles, or sebaceous glands [2]. Cervical dermoid cysts represent only 20% of head and neck dermoids [1]. Cervical dermoids present as painless superficial subcutaneous masses in the anterior neck and usually move with the skin. They can be close to the hyoid and move with swallowing or tongue protrusion leading to confusion with thyroglossal duct cysts. They gradually increase in size over time because of accumulation of sebum. Infection is rare, but the cysts can rupture and present with granulomatous inflammation. They are often diagnosed before the patient is 3 years old [1].

Evaluation begins with history and physical examination, but can be augmented with ultrasonography to delineate the depth of the lesion and its relationship to the hyoid bone. If the lesion is inflamed, fine needle aspirate may be helpful to distinguish between a ruptured dermoid cyst and an infected thyroglossal duct cyst. If the lesion is symptomatic, enlarging, or has ruptured, surgical excision is recommended. Complete simple excision is usually adequate, but if it is attached to the hyoid bone a Sistrunk procedure should be performed to prevent inadequate excision of an atypical thyroglossal duct cyst [19]. Rate of recurrence is increased by incomplete resection or intraoperative rupture [2].

Teratomas differ from dermoid cysts in that they contain all three germ layers. Head and neck lesions compose less than 2% of teratomas, with the most common sites being the nasopharynx and neck. They develop during the second trimester and present as rapidly expanding lateral or midline neck masses. They may be diagnosed by prenatal ultrasonography, with 30% accompanied by polyhydramnios because of esophageal obstruction [1]. If the diagnosis is known before delivery, cesarean section is recommended. Although the lesions may initially be asymptomatic, rapid growth may eventually lead to dysphagia and respiratory distress. Eighty percent of infants who have neonatal teratomas may die if untreated [1]. Ultrasound, CT, or MRI may be helpful in evaluating these lesions. Some neonates may require intubation or even extracorporeal membrane oxygenation if the lesion has caused pulmonary hypoplasia. Complete surgical excision is the treatment of choice once the airway has been stabilized. Malignancy has not been reported in pediatric cervical teratomas, so all critical structures in the neck should be spared [1]. Malignant cervical teratomas have

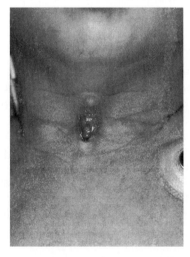

Fig. 11. Congenital midline cervical cleft. (*From* Foley DS, Fallat ME. Thyroglossal duct and other congenital midline cervical anomalies. Semin Pediatr Surg 2006;15:70–5; with permission.)

been found in adults and require aggressive treatment because they can spread by hematogenous and lymphatic routes and carry a poor prognosis.

Midline cervical clefts

Midline cervical clefts are rare congenital cervical anomalies. They are present at birth as a cutaneous ulceration with overhanging skin or cartilaginous tag in the anterior lower midline of the neck (Fig. 11). There is often a sinus tract that extends downward from the skin and may connect to the sternum or mandible or end in a blind pouch. The embryologic origin is unknown but is believed to be a "mesodermal fusion abnormality involving the paired branchial arches during gestational weeks 3 and 4" [2]. Fibrous tissue with interwoven skeletal muscle is present. Most cases are sporadic, but can be associated with other cleft abnormalities of the tongue, lower lip, or mandible. If untreated, some clefts can result in neck contractures or growth deformities of the mandible or sternum. Early surgical excision at the time of diagnosis is recommended, therefore, with complete excision of the skin lesion and the subcutaneous sinus to reduce the rate of recurrence. This excision can usually be accomplished by stair-step incisions, but if more complicated may require a series of Z-plasty incisions to improve the cosmetic and functional result [2].

References

[1] Enepekides DJ. Management of congenital anomalies of the neck. Facial Plast Surg Clin North Am 2001;9:131–45.

[2] Foley DS, Fallat ME. Thyroglossal duct and other congenital midline cervical anomalies. Semin Pediatr Surg 2006;15:70–5.

[3] Perez-Martinez A, Bento-Bravo L, Martinez-Bermejo MA, et al. An intra-thyroid thyroglossal duct cyst. Eur J Pediatr Surg 2005;15:428–30.

[4] Mohan PS, Chokshi RA, Moser RL, et al. Thyroglossal duct cysts: a consideration in adults. Am Surg 2005;71(6):508–11.

[5] Pinczower E, Crockett DM, Atkinson JB, et al. Preoperative thyroid scanning in presumed thyroglossal duct cysts. Arch Otolaryngol Head Neck Surg 1992;118:985–8.

[6] Peretz A, Lieberman E, Kapelsuhnik J, et al. Thyroglossal duct carcinoma in children: case presentation and review of the literature. Thyroid 2004;14:777–85.

[7] Ostlie DJ, Burjonrappa SC, Synder CI, et al. Thyroglossal duct infections and surgical outcomes. J Pediatr Surg 2004;39:396–9.

[8] Waldhausen JHT. Branchial cleft and arch anomalies in children. Semin Pediatr Surg 2006; 15:64–9.

[9] D'Souza AR, Uppal HS, De R, et al. Updating concepts of first brachial cleft defects: a literature review. Int J Pediatr Otolaryngol 2002;62:103–9.

[10] Shrime M, Kacker A, Bent J, et al. Fourth branchial complex anomalies: a case series. Int J Pediatr Otolaryngol 2003;67:1227–33.

[11] Roback SA, Telander RL. Thyroglossal duct cysts and branchial cleft anomalies. Semin Pediatr Surg 1994;3:142–6.

[12] O'Mara W, Amedee R. Anomalies of the branchial apparatus. J La State Med Soc 1998;150: 570–3.

[13] Triglia JM, Nicollas R, Ducroz V, et al. First branchial cleft anomalies. Arch Otolaryngol Head Neck Surg 1998;124:291–5.
[14] Liberman M, Kay S, Emil S, et al. Ten years experience with third and fourth branchial remnants. J Pediatr Surg 2002;37:685–90.
[15] Ford GR, Balakrishman A, Evans JN, et al. Branchial cleft and pouch anomalies. J Laryngol Otol 1992;106:137–43.
[16] Park SW, Han MH, Sung MH, et al. Neck infection associated with pyriform sinus fistula: imaging findings. AJNR Am J Neuroradiol 2000;21:817–22.
[17] Nicollas R, Ducroz V, Garabedian EN, et al. Fourth branchial pouch anomalies: a study of six cases and a review of the literature. Int J Pediatr Otorhinolaryngol 1998;44:5–10.
[18] Smith RJH, Schwartz C. Branchio-oto-renal syndrome. J Commun Disord 1998;31:411–21.
[19] Turkyilmaz Z, Sonmez K, Karabulut R, et al. Management of thyroglossal duct cysts in children. Pediatr Int 2004;46:77–80.

ELSEVIER
SAUNDERS

Otolaryngol Clin N Am
40 (2007) 177–191

OTOLARYNGOLOGIC
CLINICS
OF NORTH AMERICA

Congenital Anomalies of the Larynx

Sidrah M. Ahmad, BS, Ahmed M.S. Soliman, MD*

*Department of Otolaryngology–Head & Neck Surgery, Temple University
School of Medicine, 3400 North Broad Street, Kresge West 102,
Philadelphia, PA 19140, USA*

Congenital laryngeal anomalies are relatively rare (Fig. 1). However, they may present with life-threatening respiratory problems in the newborn period. Associated problems with phonation and swallowing may prevent a baby from thriving. Stridor is a common presenting sign in laryngeal obstruction [1]. The source of the obstruction can be suspected based on the characteristics of the stridor. Supraglottic or glottic obstruction generally present as inspiratory stridor. Biphasic stridor suggests a narrowing between the glottis and extrathoracic trachea. Turbulent airflow in the distal trachea or main bronchi can produce expiratory stridor.

Embryology

Much of our current understanding of the embryologic development of the larynx comes from the works of Tucker and colleagues [2], Zaw-Tun [3] and Hollinger and colleagues [4]. Based on the Carnegie staging system, the development of the larynx is divided into two periods: the embryonic and the fetal period [5,6]. The embryonic period comprises the first 8 weeks of intrauterine development. The larynx first appears around day 25 to 28 of gestation as an epithelial thickening along the ventral aspect of the foregut, called the respiratory primordium. As the respiratory primordium develops, the respiratory diverticulum, an outpouching of the foregut lumen, grows into it. The respiratory diverticulum develops in the area of the primitive pharyngeal floor at the level of the adult glottis. The pharyngeal floor and the primitive pharyngeal floor are divided by the primitive laryngopharynx, which develops into the adult supraglottis.

Over time, the respiratory diverticulum extends inferiorly and is separated from the developing heart and liver by the septum transversum, and

---

* Corresponding author.
E-mail address: asoliman@ent.temple.edu (A.M.S. Soliman).

doi:10.1016/j.otc.2006.10.004
oto.theclinics.com

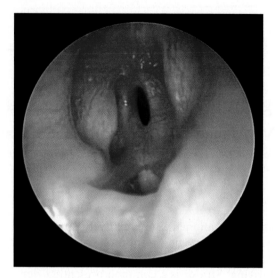

Fig. 1. Subglottic web.

from the esophagus by the tracheoesophageal septum. The tracheoesophageal septum grows in a caudal to cranial direction. If cranial advancement is impeded, a tracheolaryngeal or laryngeal cleft or tracheoesophageal fistula may form. Abnormal development of the respiratory diverticulum itself may result in tracheal agenesis, tracheal stenosis, or complete tracheal rings.

Obliteration of the ventral lumen of the primitive laryngopharynx gives rise to the epithelial lamina. Located dorsal to the epithelial lamina is the pharyngoglottic duct, which develops into the interarytenoid notch and posterior glottis. Located anterior to the epithelial lamina is the laryngeal cecum, which becomes the laryngeal vestibule. The epithelial lamina then recanalizes to allow for the laryngeal cecum and the pharyngoglottic duct to unite. Failure to recanalize may result in laryngeal webs or stenosis.

During the fetal period, the vocal processes form from the arytenoids, the goblet cells and submucosal glands develop, and the epiglottic cartilage matures into a fibrocartilaginous structure [7]. The fetal period lasts approximately 32 weeks. Toward the end of gestation, the cricoid cartilage changes from interstitial to perichondrial growth.

Anomalies

Laryngomalacia

Laryngomalacia is the leading cause of stridor in infants, and accounts for approximately 60% to 75% of congenital laryngeal anomalies (Fig. 2) [8–11]. Laryngomalacia was first described by Jackson and Jackson in 1942 as a disorder in which supraglottic tissue collapses onto the glottis

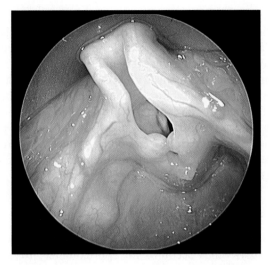

Fig. 2. Combined laryngomalacia.

upon inspiration [12]. This disorder typically produces a high-pitched, inspiratory stridor during the first 2 weeks of extrauterine life and spontaneously resolves by age 12 to 24 months [8–11,14,15]. In severe cases of laryngomalacia, a child may suffer from apneic events, pulmonary hypertension, or failure to thrive. In such cases, surgical intervention is warranted, including supraglottoplasty, division of the aryepiglottic folds, or epiglottopexy [9–11].

Laryngomalacia is diagnosed by flexible fiberoptic endoscopy [8]. It is classified as type 1, type 2, or type 3, based on patterns of supraglottic collapse [8–10]. In type 1 laryngomalacia, redundant supraglottic mucosa prolapses; type 2 is characterized by shortened aryepiglottic folds; and type 3 displays posterior displacement of the epiglottis.

Type 1 laryngomalacia is treated with supraglottoplasty, in which redundant epiglottic, aryepiglottic folds, or arytenoids mucosa is excised [8]. This procedure may be performed using microsurgical instruments, a carbon dioxide (CO_2) laser, or the laryngeal microdebrider [10–11,13,16] CO_2 laser supraglottoplasty allows for precise excision of the redundant tissue, with minimal bleeding [11,13]. Endoscopic supraglottoplasty with a laryngeal microdebrider allows for the negative pressures associated with inspiration to be simulated by suction, and thus allows the surgeon to better visualize and excise the redundant tissue [16]. Type 2 laryngomalacia is treated best with an incision in the aryepiglottic folds to allow expansion of the airway [11]. Typically, a wedge is excised from the aryepiglottic folds; however, Loke and colleagues [17] demonstrated that a simple incision dividing the aryepiglottic folds is sufficient for alleviation of airway obstruction. The division of the aryepiglottic folds may be performed with microlaryngeal scissors or the CO_2 laser. Type 3 laryngomalacia can be treated effectively by way of epiglottopexy, in which the epiglottis is tacked to the base of the tongue, thereby rectifying the posterior displacement of the epiglottis [11]. Not all cases can be classified easily into a single category; thus, a combination of surgical options may be used for treatment.

Gastroesophageal reflux disease (GERD) has been associated with laryngomalacia [8,10,18]. It is unclear whether GERD causes laryngomalacia by inducing diffuse edema of the larynx, or laryngomalacia causes GERD by inducing high negative intrapleural pressure and thereby preventing the lower esophageal sphincter from functioning properly. In either case, it is beneficial to treat laryngomalacia patients suffering from GERD with anti-reflux measures.

Congenital vocal fold immobility

The second most common congenital laryngeal disorder is vocal fold movement disorder, which accounts for approximately 10% to 20% of all congenital laryngeal anomalies [8,19,20] Unilateral vocal fold immobility (VFI) typically presents with a weak, breathy cry, feeding difficulties, and aspiration [8,20] Bilateral VFI, the less common of the two, typically presents with biphasic stridor and a preserved cry [20]. Some neonates with bilateral VFI require intubation at birth because of severe respiratory distress, whereas others have little or no airway compromise.

Most cases of VFI are idiopathic in nature; however, the disorder may result from birth trauma, central or peripheral nervous system anomalies, or cardiovascular anomalies [20]. Central and peripheral nervous system disorders may result in unilateral or bilateral VFI [15,20]. Central nervous system disorders associated with VFI include brain stem or cerebral dysgenesis, hydrocephalus, encephalocele, leukodystrophy, meningomyelocele, hydrocephalus, spina bifida, cerebral palsy, and Arnold-Chiari malformation (ACM). Though ACM is associated most commonly with bilateral VFI, it can cause unilateral VFI [20]. Peripheral nervous system disorders associated with VFI include myasthenia gravis, fascioscapulohumeral myopathy, and spinal muscular atrophy. Cardiovascular anomalies associated with VFI include ventricular septal defect, Tetralogy of Fallot, cardiomegaly, Ortner syndrome, vascular rings, double aortic arch, and patent ductus arteriosus [15,20].

Hereditary bilateral VFI has been identified [20]. In 1978, Mace and colleagues [21] suggested autosomal dominant inheritance in some cases of bilateral VFI. In 2001, Manaligod and colleagues [22] identified chromosome 6q16 as the locus responsible for hereditary bilateral VFI. No genetic cause has been identified in the case of unilateral VFI [20].

Endoscopy is essential in evaluating the airway and vocal fold motion [15,20,23]. A combination of awake flexible laryngoscopy and rigid bronchoscopy under anesthesia has been advocated [15,20]. In a complete evaluation, the arytenoids should be palpated to determine the mobility of the cricoarytenoid joints [20,24]. Adjunctive tests include video contrast esophagography to assess swallowing function, and laryngeal electromyography to help differentiate between vocal fold fixation and paralysis [15,20,24,25]. Infants with bilateral, vocal fold movement impairment should undergo cranial imaging (CT, ultrasonography, or MRI) to rule out brainstem pathology, a careful physical examination of the neck, and a chest radiograph or CT to look for mediastinal pathology.

In patients who have VFI secondary to another medical disorder, the underlying cause should be treated [15,20]. In most cases, idiopathic congenital VFI spontaneously resolves within the first 6 to 12 months of life, although recovery has been documented up to 11 years later [1,20,23]. As such, treatment of neonates should be conservative. In cases of significant airway compromise, a tracheotomy may be required until spontaneous recovery of vocal fold motion occurs [8,20,23].

In patients who have unilateral VFI and are prone to aspiration, a nasogastric feeding tube or gastrostomy tube may be placed to ensure adequate nutritional intake [19]. Injection medialization of the paralyzed vocal fold with absorbable gelatin sponge (Gelfoam) or collagen is also effective in reducing aspiration in older children [1,20,23]. Type I thyroplasty offers an alternative to injection medialization [1,20]. Much controversy surrounds the use of these procedures in the pediatric population. In infants and young children, medialization of a paretic vocal fold may worsen in the airway. The effects of medialization laryngoplasty on the growing laryngeal framework are unknown [20].

In patients who have bilateral VFI, treatment options include vocal fold lateralization, partial cordectomy, arytenoidectomy by way of endoscopic or external approach, and expansion of the cricoid cartilage by way of anterior cricoid split (ACS) with graft placement [1,8,26]. Friedman and colleagues [26] have demonstrated the use of the CO_2 laser to perform a posterior transverse partial cordectomy in which a portion of the posterior vocal fold is removed after releasing the vocal ligament and vocalis muscle from the arytenoid cartilage. The CO_2 laser has been used successfully for this procedure in the adult population for many years. It may be a viable option in children with significantly compromised airways and little or no prospect for the return of adequate vocal fold function.

Laryngeal cysts

Laryngeal cysts present with variable degrees of airway obstruction, hoarseness, and dysphagia [27–29]. DeSanto and colleagues [30] classified laryngeal cysts as saccular, ductal, or thyroid cartilage foraminal cysts. In 1997, Arens and colleagues [31] created a new classification system in which the location of the cyst and histomorphology were taken into consideration. In this classification system, laryngeal cysts were classified as congenital, retention, or inclusion cysts.

Recently, Forte and colleagues [28] proposed a new classification system for congenital laryngeal cysts in an attempt to guide treatment based on classification. In this system, classification is based on the extent of the cyst and the embryologic tissue of origin. Cysts confined to the larynx and consisting of only endodermal elements are classified as type I and can be completely excised endoscopically. Cysts with extralaryngeal extension are classified as type II and typically, for complete excision, an open approach is used. Type II cysts are subdivided further into type IIa and IIb. Type IIa cysts originate embryologically from endodermal elements, whereas type IIb cysts originate from both endodermal and mesodermal elements, as seen in laryngotracheal duplication cysts or diverticula. The authors use the DeSanto classification system in the later discussion.

Saccular cysts

The saccule is a membranous pouch located between the ventricular fold and the inner surface of the thyroid cartilage [32]. The normal mucous membrane surface of the saccule is covered with openings to 60 or 70 mucous glands. Compression of the saccule by surrounding muscles allows these mucous secretions to lubricate the surfaces of the vocal folds.

Saccular cysts result from obstruction of the laryngeal saccule orifice in the ventricle, with resultant mucus retention in the saccule (Fig. 3) [28]. Although saccular cysts may be identified radiographically, endoscopy is the gold standard for diagnosis [23]. Endoscopic evaluation reveals a cystic lesion containing thick, mucoid fluid emanating from behind the aryepiglottic fold in the case of lateral cysts, or from the ventricles and protruding into the laryngeal lumen in the case of anterior cysts [8,33]. Needle aspiration may be useful in

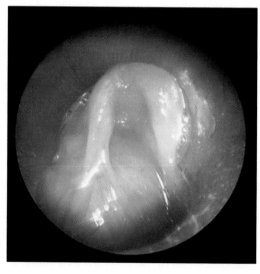

Fig. 3. Saccular cyst.

diagnosing the lesion, but drainage of the cyst offers only temporary treatment [23,33]. Marsupialization may be adequate for the treatment of small saccular cysts. However, in the case of recurrence or large cysts, endoscopic or open excision of the cyst is required to remove the cystic tissue completely [5,25].

Vallecular cysts

Most neonates with vallecular cysts (Fig. 4) present with stridor within the first few weeks of birth [1]. Other symptoms include cough, feeding difficulties, cyanotic episodes, and failure to thrive. Among the many theories regarding the pathogenesis of vallecular cysts, the most likely states that they are the result of an obstruction of mucosal glands located at the base of the tongue [29]. Mucosal secretions from glands surrounding the cyst cause the cyst to increase in size.

CT may be useful in demonstrating the location and extent of the cyst; [29] however, endoscopy is important in accurately diagnosing vallecular cysts and ruling out other vallecular lesions such as dermoids, teratomas, lingual thyroid, lymphangiomas, or hemangiomas [1,29]. Endoscopic evaluation reveals a smooth mass localized in the vallecular space. Radionuclide thyroid scans might help to localize functioning thyroid tissue.

Definitive treatment of vallecular cysts consists of endoscopic excision or marsupialization [1,29]. Aspiration of the cyst may be useful in securing a tenuous airway, but uniformly leads to recurrence.

Thyroglossal duct cysts

Although they are found most commonly in the neck, thyroglossal duct cysts may also present in the vallecula and cause airway obstruction [1].

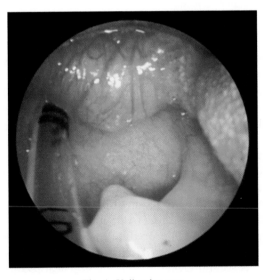

Fig. 4. Vallecular cyst.

These cysts are lined by pseudostratified ciliated or squamous epithelium. Adjacent stroma contain mucous glands and thyroid follicles. Histologic identification of thyroid follicles helps to differentiate thyroglossal duct cysts from vallecular cysts.

Ductal cysts

Cysts resulting from an obstruction of submucosal mucous glands are referred to as ductal cysts [1,29]. These cysts commonly occur in the vallecula and vocal folds. As with other cysts, treatment consists of marsupialization or complete excision of the lesion.

Laryngoceles

Laryngoceles are the result of an abnormal dilation of the laryngeal saccule [23]. Unlike saccular cysts, laryngoceles communicate with the laryngeal lumen [23,34,35]. Laryngoceles intermittently fill with air and expand the saccule, which impinges on the laryngeal lumen, causing airway obstruction and a weak cry. The dilated saccule may enlarge and extend into the neck through the thyrohyoid membrane.

Radiographic studies may reveal an air-containing sac in the aryepiglottic fold or out into the neck. Endoscopic evaluation is important to rule out other laryngeal lesions, such as laryngeal duplication cysts, hamartomas, choristomas, and teratomas that may have similar appearances and presentations [27,34]. Endoscopic marsupialization is sufficient to control most internal laryngoceles [23,28,35]. When there is an external component, an open approach may be necessary to remove the lesion completely [35].

Laryngeal atresia and stenosis

Laryngeal atresia

Laryngeal atresia is an extremely rare condition that results from the failure of the larynx and trachea to recanalize during embryogenesis [5]. Typical presentation at birth is severe respiratory distress despite strong respiratory effort. Laryngeal atresia can be diagnosed prenatally based on ultrasonographic evaluation, by identifying the signs of congenital high airway obstruction syndrome (CHAOS), such as hyperechogenic enlarged lungs, a flattened or inverted diaphragm, a fluid-filled, dilated airway distal to the obstruction, fetal hydrops, and polyhydramnios [36–38]. Color flow Doppler ultrasonography is useful in localizing the level of the obstruction by detecting the absence of flow in the trachea during fetal breathing.

An emergent tracheotomy is required immediately upon birth to secure an airway. Prenatal diagnosis of CHAOS allows for the use of the ex utero intrapartum treatment (EXIT) procedure to evaluate and secure the airway at birth [36,37]. In this procedure, placental support is maintained after birth until the airway is secure. Generally, laryngotracheal reconstruction is performed at a later stage [5,6].

Associated anomalies include tracheoesophageal fistula, esophageal atresia, urinary tract abnormalities, limb defects, encephalocele, horseshoe kidney, and low-set ears [5,37]. In neonates with an associated tracheoesophageal fistula, it is possible to secure the airway temporarily by way of esophageal intubation.

Congenital subglottic stenosis

Congenital subglottic stenosis is diagnosed when there is a narrowing of the laryngeal lumen in the cricoid region and no history of intubation or surgical trauma. Most investigators consider a diameter of less than 4 mm in a full-term newborn and 3 mm in a premature infant to be insufficient [5,6]. However, some investigators quote a diameter of less than 3.5 mm in a newborn [1,8]. Congenital subglottic stenosis was described by Holinger in 1954 as a malformation of the cricoid cartilage [39]. The transverse and anteroposterior luminal diameters at the midportion of the cricoid cartilage are normally equal [1]. Holinger described an elliptic cricoid cartilage in which the transverse diameter was significantly smaller [40].

Congenital subglottic stenosis can be classified as either membranous or cartilaginous [5]. Membranous stenosis is the more common and milder type of congenital stenosis. It results from submucosal gland hypoplasia with excessive fibrous connective tissue. Cartilaginous stenosis has three common variants: an abnormally shaped cricoid cartilage with lateral shelves, and an elliptic shape, or a normally shaped cricoid cartilage with a decreased diameter.

Usually, congenital subglottic stenosis is diagnosed in the first few months of life. Symptoms of subglottic stenosis range from mild dyspnea to severe airway obstruction [5,23]. Stridor tends to be biphasic or primarily inspiratory in nature. In mild cases, symptoms manifest only during respiratory tract infections, when edema and thickened secretions further compromise the airway. Recurrent or persistent croup is a typical finding in children with subglottic stenosis. Children with Down syndrome have a high incidence of congenital airway narrowing [5]. Often, these children are asymptomatic but prove difficult to intubate for anesthesia.

The severity of the subglottic stenosis usually is determined by the Myer-Cotton grading system [1,5]. Endotracheal tubes of various sizes are placed sequentially, with the second graduated mark at the level of the vocal cords. The endotracheal tube, which results in a leak pressure of less than 30 cm H_2O, is considered to be the individual's tube size. The patient's tube size and age are compared with established norms and a grade is assigned.

Plain radiographs are of limited value in assessing the subglottis [8,23]. Anterior-posterior cervical airway radiographs reveal a classic hourglass narrowing at the level of the subglottis [8].

Congenital subglottic stenosis becomes less critical as the larynx grows. Symptoms resolve by a few years of age in most cases [5,8]. Thus, for grade I stenosis, a watch and wait approach is deemed appropriate [1]. For more severe cases of congenital subglottic stenosis, surgical intervention may be necessary [1,5,25]. Fewer than 50% of children require a tracheotomy and most who do can be decannulated once the airway improves sufficiently [5]. Other surgical options, such as anterior laryngotracheal decompression or reconstruction, have been advocated to avoid the potential complications of tracheotomy, including an increased risk of infection, accidental decannulation, tracheotomy tube plugging, and retardation in speech and language development [1,5,8,23,41]. Dilation and endoscopic laser surgery are ineffective, particularly in cartilaginous stenosis [1,23].

Cotton and Seid described the ACS procedure as an alternative to tracheotomy in 1980 [42]. The success rate of this procedure for the treatment of neonates with subglottic stenosis ranges from 58% to 100%, with few complications. The ACS procedure entails the division of the cricoid cartilage, the first two tracheal rings, and the caudal thyroid cartilage in the midline. In 1991, Richardson and colleagues [43] demonstrated that the use of a rib cartilaginous graft in conjunction with ACS resulted in improved efficacy. Since then, auricular cartilage, hyoid bone, and thyroid alar cartilage all have been used to expand the narrowed subglottis [44–46].

Subglottic hemangiomas

Hemangiomas are congenital vascular lesions that undergo rapid growth in the first months after birth [8,47,48]. Their size stabilizes between 12 and 18 months. Finally, most hemangiomas involute, generally by 5 years of age [47].

Congenital subglottic hemangiomas are rare, but potentially fatal, lesions (Fig. 5). They account for 1.5% of congenital laryngeal abnormalities [1,8,49]. They have a female/male ratio of 2:1 [41,50,51]. Presentation may

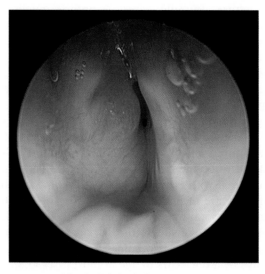

Fig. 5. Subglottic hemangioma.

be similar to that of subglottic stenosis, with recurrent croup and biphasic stridor [8,37]. Other symptoms may include a barking cough, hoarseness, cyanosis, hemoptysis, dysphagia, and failure to thrive [8,52]. Approximately 50% of infants have cutaneous hemangiomas as well [8,50].

Hemangiomas are suspected by history, physical examination, and, typically, endoscopic appearance [8]. Plain radiographs of the neck may show asymmetric narrowing of the subglottis [52]. Flexible endoscopy may suggest the diagnosis and is useful in ruling out other laryngeal abnormalities [8]. Rigid endoscopy reveals a red-to-blue, compressible, sessile lesion that most commonly is located posterolaterally in the subglottis [47]. Histologic confirmation carries the risk of hemorrhage. Microscopically, hemangiomas are composed of small, thin-walled vessels of capillary size that are lined by a single layer of flattened or plump endothelial cells and surrounded by a discontinuous layer of pericytes and reticular fibers.

Many options are available for the treatment of subglottic hemangiomas. Traditionally, a watchful waiting approach with or without a tracheotomy has been taken [49]. A tracheotomy secures the airway until the hemangioma naturally regresses. With advances in therapy to decrease the size of the lesion, tracheotomy can be avoided and associated complications prevented [52]. Treatment options include radiation therapy, cryotherapy, sclerotherapy, alpha-2A interferon therapy, systemic or intralesional corticosteroid use, open surgical resection, and laser ablation [41,47,50,52,53].

Radiation therapy, cryotherapy, and sclerotherapy have been discontinued because of their adverse effects [41,47]. Radiation therapy was introduced first in 1919 by New and Clark [54]. The treatment showed potential. However, because of the risk of damage to normal airway mucosa and an increased risk of malignancy, the treatment was abandoned in the late 1970s [47]. Cryotherapy was used first by Schechter and Biller in 1972, with transient responses [55]. The extent of tissue damage, however, is unpredictable with this therapy and may result in subglottic stenosis [47]. As such, this therapy has fallen out of favor. Sclerotherapy has been deemed not only ineffective as a cure but also associated with complications such as hemoglobinuria, nerve injury, ulceration, and cardiovascular collapse [48]. Currently, research is being conducted to improve sclerosant agents and delivery methods that would result in greater efficacy and fewer adverse effects.

In 1994, Ohlms and colleagues [56] reported successful treatment of subglottic hemangiomas in eight patients, using interferon alpha-2a. However, this treatment option has fallen out of favor as a first line treatment because of the risk of spastic diplegia [47,48].

The use of systemic corticosteroids has been proven effective in 25% of cases [57]. A diminished rate of proliferation, softening of the tumor, and a fading of the color should occur between a few days and a few weeks of initiating therapy [47,57]. It is important to gradually taper off steroids to prevent rebound growth [47]. This method is most effective for treating small lesions;

[57] however, long-term steroid use is not without complications. Adverse effects of long-term use include Cushing's syndrome, hypertension, immune deficiency, and growth retardation [41,57]. Intralesional steroid injection has the benefits of systemic corticosteroid therapy without the adverse effects [29]. However, local steroid injection requires multiple treatments [47,57].

Open surgical resection for the treatment of subglottic hemangiomas was described first by Sharp in 1949 [58]. Currently, it is recommended for certain airway-threatening lesions, including large, obstructing hemangiomas in the proliferating phase; bilateral subglottic hemangiomas; and hemangiomas with extralaryngeal extension [41,50,51,53]. In 1974, Evans and Todd [59] described surgical excision of hemangiomas followed by laryngotracheoplasty. All three of their patients required a tracheotomy and postoperative stenting. Advances in laryngotracheoplasty procedures allow for open surgical resection to be performed, as either a single-stage procedure with short-term endotracheal intubation or as a staged procedure with delayed decannulation after the subglottis has healed completely [8,53].

CO_2 laser ablation in the treatment of subglottic hemangiomas was described by Simpson and colleagues in 1979 [60]. In 1980, Healy and colleagues [61] demonstrated the efficacy of CO_2 laser ablation with one or two applications in 11 patients. This treatment has produced mixed results, ranging from reports of earlier decannulation and low complication rates, to minimal benefits and high complication rates [47,53]. Complications include significant scar tissue and subglottic stenosis [41,47,50].

The use of the potassium-titanyl-phosphate (KTP) laser has also shown potential in the treatment of subglottic hemangiomas [47,50]. The KTP laser with a wavelength of 532 nm is absorbed preferentially by hemoglobin. Unlike CO_2 lasers, its light can be transmitted through flexible fiberscopes [50,51]. The KTP laser has significant tissue penetration and can cause thermal damage to the cricoid and tracheal cartilages [47,50,51]. In a series of six patients, Madgy and colleagues [39] reported a grade 1 subglottic stenosis in one patient after laser ablation with a KTP laser.

References

[1] Messner AH. Congenital disorders of the larynx. In: Cummings CW, editor. Otolaryngology: head & neck surgery. 4th edition. St. Louis (MO): Mosby, Inc.; 2005. p. 4223–40.
[2] Tucker GF, Tucker JA, Vidic B. Anatomy and development of the cricoid: serial-section whole organ study of perinatal larynges. Ann Otol Rhinol Laryngol 1977;86(6 Pt 1):766–9.
[3] Zaw-Tun HI. Development of congenital laryngeal atresias and clefts. Ann Otol Rhinol Laryngol 1988;97(4 Pt 1):353–8.
[4] Holinger LD, Lusk RP, Green CG. Pediatric Laryngology and Bronchoesophagology. Philadelphia: Lippincott-Raven; 1997.
[5] Hartnick CJ, Cotton RT. Syndromic and other congenital anomalies of the head and neck. Otolaryngol Clin North Am 2003;33(6):1293–308.
[6] Wyatt ME, Hartley BEJ. Laryngotracheal reconstruction in congenital laryngeal webs and atresia. Otolaryngol Head Neck Surg 2005;132(2):232–8.

[7] Manoukian BL, Tak AK. Embryology of the larynx. In: Tewfik TL, Der Kaloustian VM, editors. Congenital anomalies of the ear, nose, and throat. New York: Oxford University Press; 1997. p. 377–82.

[8] Wiatrak BJ. Congenital anomalies of the larynx and trachea. Otolaryngol Clin North Am 2000;33(1):91–110.

[9] Daniel SJ. The upper airway: congenital malformations. Paediatr Respir Rev 2006;7(Suppl 1): S260–3.

[10] Onley DR, Greinwald JH, Smith RJH, et al. Laryngomalacia and its treatment. Laryngoscope 1999;109(11):1770–5.

[11] Werner JA, Lippert BM, Dunne AA, et al. Epiglottopexy for the treatment of severe layngomalacia. Eur Arch Otorhinolaryngol 2002;259(9):459–64.

[12] Jackson C, Jackson CL. In: Diseases and Injuries of the Larynx. New York: Macmillan; 1942. p. 63–9.

[13] Senders CW, Navarrete EG. Laser supraglottoplasty for laryngomalacia: are specific anatomical defects more influential than associated anomalies on outcome? Int J Pediatr Otorhinolaryngol 2001;57(3):235–44.

[14] Sichel JY, Dangoor E, Eliashar R, et al. Management of congenital laryngeal malformations. Am J Otolaryngol 2000;21(1):22–30.

[15] Dinwiddie R. Congenital upper airway obstruction. Paediatr Respir Rev 2004;5(1):17–24.

[16] Zalzal GH, Collins WO. Microdebrider-assisted supraglottoplasty. Int J Pediatr Otorhinolaryngol 2005;69(3):305–9.

[17] Loke D, Ghosh S, Panarese A, et al. Endoscopic division of the ary-epiglottic folds in severe laryngomalacia. Int J Pediatr Otorhinolaryngol 2001;60(1):59–63.

[18] Bibi H, Khvolis E, Shoseyov D, et al. The prevalence of gastroesophageal reflux in children with tracheomalacia and laryngomalacia. Chest 2001;119(2):409–13.

[19] Patel NJ, Kerschner JE, Merati AL. The use of injectable collagen in the management of pediatric vocal unilateral fold paralysis. Int J Pediatr Otorhinolaryngol 2003;67(12): 1355–60.

[20] Parikh SR. Pediatric unilateral vocal fold immobility. Otolaryngol Clin North Am 2004; 37(1):203–15.

[21] Mace M, Williamson E, Worgan D. Autosomal dominantly inherited adductor laryngeal paralysis–a new syndrome with a suggestion of linkage to HLA. Clin Genet 1978;14(5):265–70.

[22] Manaligod JM, Skaggs J, Smith RJ. Localization of the gene for familial laryngeal abductor paralysis to chromosome 6q16. Arch Otolaryngol Head Neck Surg 2001;127(8):913–7.

[23] Holinger LD. Congenital anomalies of the larynx. In: Behrman RE, editor. Nelson textbook of pediatrics. 17th edition. Philadelphia: WB Saunders; 2004. p. 1409–10.

[24] Berkowitz RG. Laryngeal electromyography findings in idiopathic congenital bilateral vocal cord paralysis. Ann Otol Rhinol Laryngol 1996;105(3):207–12.

[25] Jacobs IN, Finkel RS. Laryngeal electromyography in the management of vocal cord mobility problems in children. Laryngoscope 2002;112(7):1243–8.

[26] Friedman EM, de Jong AL, Sulek M. Pediatric bilateral vocal fold immobility: the role of carbon dioxide laser posterior transverse partial cordectomy. Ann Otol Rhinol Laryngol 2001;110(8):723–8.

[27] Nussenbaum B, McClay JE, Timmons CF. Laryngeal duplication cyst. Arch Otolaryngol Head Neck Surg 2002;128(11):1317–20.

[28] Forte V, Fuoco G, James A. A new classification system for congenital laryngeal cysts. Laryngoscope 2004;114(6):1123–7.

[29] Hsieh WS, Yang PH, Wong KS, et al. Vallecular cyst: an uncommon cause of stridor in newborn infants. Eur J Pediatr 2000;159(1–2):79–81.

[30] DeSanto LW, Devine KD, Weiland LH. Cysts of the larynx–classification. Laryngoscope 1970;80(1):145–76.

[31] Arens C, Glanz H, Kleinsasser O. Clinical and morphological aspects of laryngeal cysts. Eur arch Otorhinolaryngol 1997;254(9–10):430–6.

[32] Gray H, Williams PL, Warwick R. Gray's Anatomy, 36th edition. Williams PL, Warwick R, editors. Philadelphia: WB Saunders; 1980. p. 1233–4.

[33] Thabet MH, Kotob H. Lateral saccular cysts of the larynx. Aetiology, diagnosis and management. J Laryngol Otol 2001;115(4):293–7.

[34] Penngings RJE, van der Hoogen FJA, Marres HA. Giant laryngoceles: a cause of upper airway obstruction. Eur Arch Otorhinolaryngol 2001;258(12):137–40.

[35] Hirvonen TP. Endoscopic CO_2 laser surgery for large internal laryngocele. ORL J Otorhinolaryngol Relat Spec 2001;63(1):58–60.

[36] Onderoglu L, Karamursel BS, Bulun A, et al. Prenatal diagnosis of laryngeal atresia. Prenat Diagn 2003;23(4):277–80.

[37] DeCou JM, Jones DC, Jacobs HD, et al. Successful ex utero intrapartum treatment (EXIT) procedure for congenital high airway obstruction syndrome (CHAOS) owing to laryngeal atresia. J Pediatr Surg 1998;33(10):1563–5.

[38] Kalache KD, Masturzo B, Scott RJ, et al. Laryngeal atresia, encephalocele, and limb deformities (LEL): a possible new syndrome. J Med Genet 2001;38(6):420–2.

[39] Holinger PH, Johnson KC, Schiller F. Congenital anomalies of the larynx. Ann Otol Rhinol Laryngol 1954;63(3):581–606.

[40] Holinger LD, Oppenheimer RW. Congenital subglottic stenosis: the elliptical cricoid cartilage. Ann Otol Rhinol Laryngol 1989;98(9):702–6.

[41] Naiman AN, Ayri S, Froehlich P. Controlled risk of stenosis after surgical excision of laryngeal hemangioma. Arch Otolaryngol Head Neck Surg 2003;129(12):1291–5.

[42] Cotton RT, Seid AB. Management of the extubation problem in the premature child: anterior cricoid split as an alternative to tracheotomy. Ann Otol Rhinol Laryngol 1980;89(6 Pt 1): 508–11.

[43] Richardson MA, Inglis AF Jr. A comparison of anterior cricoid split with and without costal cartilage graft for acquired subglottic stenosis. Int J Pediatr Otorhinolaryngol 1991;22(2): 187–93.

[44] McGuirt WF, Little JP, Healy GB. Anterior cricoid split: use of hyoid as autologous grafting material. Arch Otolaryngol Head Neck Surg 1997;123(12):1277–80.

[45] Fraga JC, Schopf L, Forte V. Thyroid alar cartilage laryngotracheal reconstruction for severe pediatric subglottic stenosis. J Pediatr Surg 2001;36(8):1258–61.

[46] Thome R, Thome DC. Posterior cricoidotomy lumen augmentation for treatment of subglottic stenosis in children. Arch Otolaryngol Head Neck Surg 1998;124(6):660–4.

[47] Rahbar R, Nicollas R, Roger G, et al. The biology and management of subglottic hemangioma: past, present, future. Laryngoscope 2004;114(11):1880–91.

[48] Buckmiller LM. Update of hemangiomas and vascular malformations. Curr Opin Otolaryngol Head Neck Surg 2004;12(6):476–87.

[49] Bitar MA, Moukarbel RV, Zalzal GH. Management of congenital subglottic hemangioma: trends and success over the past 17 years. Otolaryngol Head Neck Surg 2005; 132(2):226–31.

[50] Kacker A, April M, Ward RF. Use of potassium titanyl phosphate (KTP) laser in management of subglottic hemangiomas. Int Pediatr Otorhinolaryngol 2001;59(1):15–21.

[51] Magdy D, Ahsan S, Kest D, et al. The application of the potassium-titanyl-phosphate (KTP) laser in the management of subglottic hemangioma. Arch Otolaryngol Head Neck Surg 2001;127(1):47–50.

[52] Holinger LD. Neoplasms of the larynx, trachea, and bronchi. In: Behrman RE, editor. Nelson textbook of pediatrics. 17th edition. Philadelphia: WB Saunders; 2004. p. 1414–5.

[53] Wiatrak BJ, Reilly JS, Seid AB, et al. Open surgical excision of subglottic hemangioma in children. Int J Pediatr Otorhinolaryngol 1996;34(1–2):191–206.

[54] New GB, Clark CM. Angioma of the larynx: reports of three cases. Ann Otol Rhinol Laryngol 1919;28:1025–37.

[55] Schechter CC, Biller HF. The limitations of corticosteroid and cryotherapy for subglottic hemangiomas. Trans Am Acad Ophthalmol Otolaryngol 1972;76:1360–2.

[56] Ohlms LA, Jones DT, McGill TJ, et al. Interferon α-2A therapy for airway hemangiomas. Ann Otol Rhinol Laryngol 1994;103(1):1–8.

[57] Vijayasekaram S, White DR, Hartley BEJ, et al. Open excision of subglottic hemangiomas to avoid tracheostomy. Arch Otolaryngol Head Neck Surg 2006;132(2): 159–63.

[58] Sharp HS. Hemangioma of the trachea in an infant, successful removal. J Laryngol Otol 1949;63:413–4.

[59] Evans JN, Todd GB. Laryngo-tracheoplasty. J Laryngol Otol 1974;88(7):589–97.

[60] Simpson GT, Healy GB, McGill TJ, et al. Benign tumors and lessions of the larynx in children: surgical excision by CO_2 laser. Ann Otol Rhinol Laryngol 1979;88(4 pt 1):479–85.

[61] Healy GB, Fearon R, French T, et al. Treatment of subglottic hemangioma with the carbon dioxide laser. Laryngoscope 1980;90(5 pt 1):809–13.

ELSEVIER
SAUNDERS

Otolaryngol Clin N Am
40 (2007) 193–217

OTOLARYNGOLOGIC
CLINICS
OF NORTH AMERICA

Congenital Tracheal Anomalies

Kishore Sandu, MD*, Philippe Monnier, MD

*Department of Otorhinolaryngology, Centre Hospitalier Universitaire Vaudois,
Lausanne 1011, Switzerland*

Congenital tracheal lesions are rare, but important, causes of morbidity in infants and children. Consequently, experience in their management is limited and dispersed. Given its small diameter, the juvenile trachea is obstructed easily by various natural causes, or following a surgical intervention. One must be aware of the various causes of these conditions, their diagnostic features, and the treatment possibilities.

Embryology of the trachea

The laryngotracheal groove, or the sulcus, appears in the proximal foregut at the third week (3 mm embryo, stage10). This groove slowly progresses caudad, and the lateral ridges form the primordium of the trachea. The pulmonary primordium appears and bulges ventrally from the foregut. Complete separation of trachea and esophagus occurs by the 11 to 14 mm stage (sixth week). The tip of the tracheal primordium buds asymmetrically, left and right, at the 4 mm stage, to provide the bronchial primordia. Mesenchymal proliferation by cells lining the coelomic cavity provides the tissue from which cartilage, muscle, and connective tissue develops. Epithelial–mesenchymal interrelationships are essential for bronchial and pulmonary development to occur. The tracheal bifurcation moves downward gradually from the neck to the level of the fourth vertebra. Cartilage appears in the trachea at 10 weeks.

Failure of complete separation of the foregut into respiratory and alimentary components is the most common defect, and produces tracheoesophageal fistula (TEF). At the upper end, the larynx may fail to reopen, producing atresia (usually a fatal anomaly), or it may fail to form a complete

---

* Corresponding author.
E-mail address: kbsandu@rediffmail.com (K. Sandu).

oto.theclinics.com

posterior septum, producing a laryngotracheoesophageal cleft (LTEC). Tracheal atresia, stenosis, and TEF may occur more distally. The relatively separate processes of laryngeal development, and budding of bronchi and pulmonary development, allow for malformations of the trachea, such as agenesis and stenosis, in the presence of a normal larynx and bronchial tree.

Anatomy

The trachea occupies the anterior and middle part of the neck and penetrates into the superior mediastinum behind the sternum. It begins at the level of the cricoid cartilage and ends at the level of the sternal angle, where it divides to form the two main or, primary, bronchi. The anterior end of the trachea is at the level of the fifth thoracic vertebra, or the sternal angle. The trachea is 4 cm long in a full-term newborn infant, and 11 to 13 cm long in an adult. The diameter of the trachea is 3 to 4 mm in a full-term newborn, and 12 to 23 mm in an adult. The lateral and anterior walls of the trachea are supported by 16 to 20 horseshoe-shaped cartilages [1]. Tracheal cartilages are C-shaped hyaline cartilages. The posterior or membranous portion of the trachea is composed of the trachealis muscle, and elastic and fibrous tissue. The ratio of cartilaginous to membranous trachea normally is 4.5:1; however, this tracheal cross-section changes during breathing and coughing as a result of changes in head and neck position and intrathoracic pressure.

The trachea has two depressions: a superior depression formed by the left thyroid lobule, and an inferior depression near the bifurcation made by the aorta. The lumen of the trachea is lined by a mucous membrane consisting of a thin lamina propria and ciliated, pseudostratified columnar epithelium. The superior and inferior thyroid, thymic, and right bronchial arteries provide the arterial supply of the trachea. The veins form rings that travel along the intercartilaginous spaces and flow into the esophageal and inferior thyroid veins. Tracheal innervation comes from the vagus nerve (pulmonary plexus and laryngeal nerves) and the sympathetic nerves (cervical and dorsal ganglia).

Assessment

Clinical findings
The diagnosis of a congenital, tracheal, obstructive anomaly is based on a high degree of suspicion in infants and children with respiratory distress accompanied by retraction. The child may have a history of respiratory difficulties of lesser intensity since birth, or shortly after birth, or of repeated and stubborn respiratory infections. Strangely, dyspnea may be episodic. Cyanosis and apneic episodes may occur. In some cases, difficulty in intubation leads to the diagnosis. Often, recurrent or persistent cough and exercise intolerance are associated. See later discussion for characteristic features of each condition.

Endoscopy

Careful use of a flexible pediatric bronchoscope can clarify much about a lesion. Rigid bronchoscopy is a procedure that allows safe ventilation during inspection, but it has to be perfectly atraumatic. The bronchoscope should not be passed into a tightly stenotic lesion, to avoid edema and inflammation, which might precipitate acute obstruction. Rigid ventilating pediatric bronchoscopes can be used for bronchoscopic evaluation. However, either a flexible pediatric bronchoscope or a long telescope (outer diameter of 2 mm) allows a more distal examination. These may be inserted through a larger, rigid, ventilating bronchoscope seated proximally, or through a pediatric operating laryngoscope. Bronchoscopes should not be forced into a stenosis, nor should any attempt be made to dilate a congenital narrowing. Ventilation is maintained by the intermittent placement of an endotracheal tube or supraglottic jet ventilation when using the laryngoscope alone for exposure. The esophagoscopy demonstrates esophageal malformations or external (often vascular) compressions. TEFs are found in the membranous wall of the trachea. Instillation of methylene blue saline into the esophagus by way of a high-placed nasogastric tube may identify a small H-type fistula conclusively.

Imaging

CT and MRI provide precise information about the cross-sectional area and extent of lesions, with three-dimensional reconstruction available. They also help in a complete mediastinal and pulmonary evaluation, which may aid in the diagnosis of associated congenital malformations. A spiral CT, because of its short duration, does not require sedation in infants. MRI offers similar information and is useful especially to delineate associated cardiovascular anomalies. Echocardiography allows a good cardiovascular evaluation, but it is often complemented by cardiac catheterization in those patients who are to undergo surgery. Angiography is also used less often, but is still the "gold standard" for precise and complete delineation of vascular anomalies [2].

Tracheal agenesis/atresia

Tracheal agenesis is a rare congenital anomaly that is not compatible with prolonged life, even with current medical technology. Its incidence is reported to be less than 1:50,000, with a male predominance [3]. The disorder was first described in 1900 by Payne, after the death of an infant on whom a tracheotomy had been attempted [4]. The absence of a trachea was noted on postmortem examination. Diagnosis can be made if the neonate presents with respiratory distress at birth, is unable to produce an audible cry in spite of an obvious physical effort, and cannot be intubated but shows some improvement when ventilated by bag and mask. An accidental esophageal intubation may improve the respiratory status temporarily if a TEF is present. In 1962, Floyd [4] proposed an anatomic classification of this malformation (Fig. 1). Type I is atresia of part of the trachea with a normal but short distal trachea, normal bronchi, and a TEF. This type makes up approximately 20% of the malformations. Sixty percent of the reported cases are type II, where there is complete tracheal atresia but normal bifurcation and bronchi. Type III, accounting for 20% of cases, has no trachea and the bronchi arise directly from the esophagus [4].

Kluth and colleagues [5] showed that the esophagus and trachea develop as the foregut decreases in size by infolding without formation of a fused septum. They proposed that tracheal atresia with fistula may result from a ventral deformation of the foregut and a concomitant dorsal dislocation of the tracheoesophageal space. Baarsma and colleagues [6] suggested that this condition should be suspected if the antenatal ultrasound examination shows abnormal fetal breathing movement. Antenatal ultrasonography may show bilateral uniform hyperechoic lungs and ascites if the trachea or larynx is obstructed completely. The inspissated lung secretions cause overdistension of the lungs. Inversion or flattening of the diaphragm can occur. Contiguous compression of the fetal heart results in low-output heart failure. In the presence of an esophageal fistula, the lungs do not become enlarged because fluid escapes through the fistula into the gastrointestinal tract. Color flow Doppler ultrasonographic findings may show an absence of blood flow at the laryngeal level [5]. The most common variant has normal bronchi communicating centrally to the esophagus.

Other congenital anomalies are common in these patients. Fonkalsrud and colleagues described a newborn who survived for a short time by using the esophagus as an airway [7]. A major bronchus may also communicate directly with the esophagus while the balance of the lung is served by anomalous bronchi from a partly stenotic trachea. Microgastria is a common

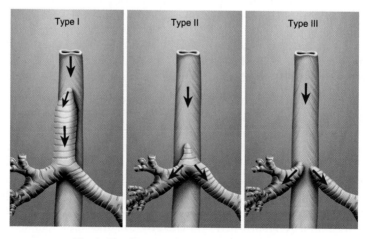

Fig. 1. Floyd's classification of tracheal agenesis.

concomitant feature. A systematic surgical approach to these anomalies does not exist, doubtless because of their rarity and variability, and the complexity of the defect [8]. Hiyama and colleagues treated one of their two infant patients successfully with the following procedures: gastrostomy and abdominal esophageal banding, translaryngeal and esophageal ventilation by endotracheal tube, tracheostomy and later T tube, pharyngeal sump drainage followed by establishment of cervical esophagostomy (proximal tracheal segment present), and esophageal reconstruction by colonic interposition at age 3 years [7].

The survival of infants with tracheal agenesis is rare, and correction is very difficult. Short-term survival may be possible if there is a fistulous connection between the esophagus and bronchus. So far, 11 cases with varying degrees of tracheal agenesis have been resuscitated and treated with various palliative and tracheal reconstructive procedures. Published reports show long-term survival of three of them [3,9]. Attempts at using the esophagus as an air conduit are only temporary, but may allow sufficient time for the diagnosis to be confirmed. It is hoped that the use of tissue-engineered cartilage may improve the outcome of affected babies without other major associated congenital anomalies.

Tracheobronchomalacia

In the pediatric age group, primary or secondary tracheobronchomalacia (TBM) is the most common cause of significant airway collapse with resultant obstruction. These problems often present difficult management issues. Various underlying pathologies may lead to increased resistance in air flow and hence, increased work of breathing. Mucociliary clearance can also be impaired causing various sequelae. In most children with TBM, the condition is self-limited, with resolution occurring within 1 to 2 years. Patients who have dying spells, recurrent pneumonia, or those who cannot be weaned from long-term ventilation may require more permanent management. TBM is a rare condition of infancy and childhood, characterized by abnormal compliance of the tracheobronchial tree [10–12]. Occasionally, TBM is an isolated lesion (primary TBM). More commonly, however, the condition is associated with other congenital abnormalities (Box 1, Figs. 2 and 3), including esophageal atresia and TEF. TBM may also be secondary to extrinsic compression from vascular structures or soft tissue masses. Rarely, a primary disorder of collagen-like dyschondroplasia or polychondritis may lead to TBM.

Pathophysiology

In laminar airflow, resistance is inversely proportional to the fourth power of the radius. Thus, even small changes in airway caliber can have dramatic effects on airway resistance. In a normal airway, a stiff cartilaginous

---

Box 1. Secondary causes of tracheobronchomalacia

1. *Esophageal atresia with TEF*
2. *Extrinsic compression*
    Vascular causes (innominate artery, aortic arch ring,
       pulmonary artery sling, aberrant right subclavian)
    Cardiac causes (enlarged left atrium, enlarged pulmonary
       arteries, enlarged pulmonary veins)
    Cysts (lymphatic malformations, thymic cysts, bronchogenic
       cysts)
    Mediastinal neoplasm (teratoma, lymphoma, neuroblastoma)
    Infection (abscess)
3. *Prolonged Intubation*
4. *Chondrodysplasias*
5. *Posttraumatic result (or following tracheoplasty)*

---

framework maintains patency, despite changing intrathoracic pressures during the respiratory cycle. During expiration, positive intrathoracic pressure is transmitted to the intrathoracic airways and causes a physiologic narrowing. In patients who have TBM, the abnormally compliant tracheobronchial

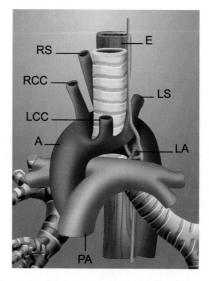

Fig. 2. Principal vascular rings that may cause extrinsic tracheal compression. A, aorta; E, esophagus; LA, ligamentum arteriosum; LCC, left common carotid artery; LS, left subclavian artery; PA, pulmonary artery; RCC, right common carotid artery; RS, right subclavian artery; V, vagus nerve.

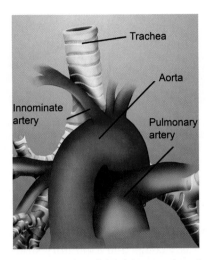

Fig. 3. Innominate artery compression of the right anterolateral aspect of the trachea.

cartilages are not able to resist increased intrathoracic pressure, leading to a collapse of the airway in the anteroposterior direction. This condition is aggravated during forced expiration and coughing, and during the Valsalva's maneuver, where the intrathoracic pressures are even higher. Also, compression by surrounding structures, anteriorly by the aorta and posteriorly by the esophagus, adds to airway collapsibility.

Pathology

In TBM patients, the tracheal cartilage is deficient or malformed, with a decreased ratio of cartilage to muscle (Fig. 4). Pathologic examination of major malacic segments reveals a decrease in the amount, size, and thickness of cartilaginous plates. Immaturity of major airway cartilage is thought to cause primary TBM. Secondary TBM likely occurs to some degree in all children with esophageal atresia. It has been postulated that an in utero tracheal compression forms a dilated esophageal pouch, leading to abnormal development. An associated loss of intratracheal pressure through a TEF may cause an additional collapsibility. Extrinsic tracheal compression is associated with tracheal cartilage abnormalities, such as hypoplasia, dysplasia, or a deficiency in the normal cartilaginous framework. Usually, a reduction in the amount of tracheal cartilage is combined with an increased width of membranous trachea in patients who have TBM. This combination of shortened, weaker tracheal rings and wider, posterior, membranous trachea results in a loss of the classic (cross-sectional) "D" configuration of the trachea. The trachea becomes compressed in the anteroposterior plane, and, in some segments, weakened cartilage is fractured into two to four pieces.

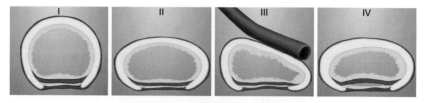

Fig. 4. Axial sections of the trachea. (*I*) normal tracheal anatomy. The ratio of the cartilaginous trachea to the posterior membranous trachea is 4/5:1. (*II*) Primary tracheomalacia; the ratio is 2/3:1. (*III*) Secondary tracheomalacia caused by an extrinsic pressure. The membranous trachea is widened. (*IV*) Tracheomalacia associated with TEF.

Signs and symptoms

Symptoms of TBM can manifest at birth, but often are evident only after 2 months of age. A brassy cough and expiratory stridor are the most common symptoms. This cough likely is caused by the abutment of the anterior and posterior walls of the trachea, which results in vibrations during cough. The most serious symptoms are dying spells or death attacks. These spells usually occur during feeding, or within 10 minutes of a meal. Patients become cyanotic and apneic, and often lose general muscle tone, which is believed to be caused by esophageal dilatation by a food bolus compressing the malacic segment from behind. If the feeding is not stopped, the symptoms can progress, leading to cardiorespiratory arrest. Respiratory infections are seen commonly in children with TBM. Respiratory secretions accumulate in distal airways because of airway collapse at the end of expiration, and may cause recurrent pneumonias.

Treatment options

In many children with TBM, intervention is not necessary. As the child grows, the tracheal cartilage strengthens and stiffens, and the symptoms often resolve by age 1 to 2 years in children with mild-to-moderate TBM. Therefore, conservative therapy in milder cases is preferred, and includes the treatment of respiratory infections, humidified oxygen therapy, and pulmonary physiotherapy. For children who do not recover spontaneously, or who have life-threatening symptoms, various treatment options are available.

The treatment of TBM has advanced in the last 3 decades. In the past, the mainstay of therapy in patients who had severe TBM was tracheotomy and long-term mechanical ventilation. Pioneering physicians recognized early that standard tracheotomy tubes were not always long enough to stent the involved segment of the trachea. Physicians developed elongated tracheotomy tubes, or advanced thin-walled tubes through a standard tracheotomy, to mechanically stent the distal trachea. The problems with this approach included the need to change the length of the tube as the child grew, recurrent bronchospasm, the negation of the glottic mechanism of in-creasing intratracheal pressure, and difficult decannulation. In addition, chronic tracheotomy produces some tracheal injury and predisposes one to recurrent infections, which has spurred the search for alternatives. The percentage of infants and children who still require tracheotomy for TBM varies from 12% to 62% [13]. Jacobs and colleagues [13] reviewed 50 cases of TBM, and reported that tracheotomy was required in 75% of premature infants and in 39% of full-term infants. Of those, 71% were able to undergo decannulation after an average of 30 months, without further intervention.

Continuous positive airway pressure (CPAP) is an effective treatment for infants with moderate to severe TBM [14]. Bronchoscopy and fluoroscopy have shown that CPAP maintains airway patency during tidal breathing. By creating a "pneumatic stent," CPAP prevents the collapse of the airway throughout the respiratory cycle. Tidal-breathing, flow-volume measure-ments have been used to evaluate the changes in airway obstruction with the use of CPAP. However, CPAP has some disadvantages [13], including a lag in the commencement of oral feedings, retardation of speech and lan-guage, and potential developmental delay. Depending on the estimated du-ration of treatment, CPAP can be considered a primary treatment, or an adjuvant to other therapies. In patients who have the most severe forms of TBM, or who present with life-threatening symptoms, surgical interven-tion may be necessary. Indications for surgery include recurrent pneumonia, intermittent respiratory obstruction, and the inability to extubate the airway [12]. Dying spells [12] are an indication for continued hospitalization and de-finitive surgical intervention.

Gross and colleagues were the first of many investigators to describe the use of aortopexy specifically for treating TBM caused by a vascular anom-aly. In this procedure, the ascending aorta is approached, traditionally through a right-sided anterior thoracotomy at the third intercostal space, or through alternative routes [15]. Traction on the sutures placed in the wall of the aorta juxtaposes it to the undersurface of the sternum, which also pulls the anterior wall of the trachea forward. This mechanical fixation of the aorta widens the anteroposterior dimensions of the trachea, and pre-vents collapse. Aortopexy is not always successful in relieving the collapse and therefore, additional surgical approaches have been devised.

External splinting with autologous materials, most commonly a resected rib, and prosthetic materials, such as silastic, membrane-reinforced, crystal-line polypropylene and high-density polyethylene (Marlex, Phillips Petro-leum, Bartlesville, Oklahoma) mesh, have been used to support the flaccid trachea [16]. Support can be provided either by suturing a rigid support di-rectly to the membranous trachea through a posterolateral right thoracot-omy or by wrapping the supporting material around three quarters of the tracheal circumference through an anterior cervical or median sternot-omy approach. Hagl and colleagues [16] described bronchoscopically guided, external tracheobronchial suspension within a ring-reinforced

polytetrafluoroethylene prosthesis, which immediately relieved severe malacia of the trachea or main bronchi in infants without necessitating resection.
In animal studies and in limited human studies, this procedure did not affect
the growth of the trachea adversely. However, it is an invasive procedure
that may not treat distal bronchial lesions adequately and may not be
well-tolerated by patients who have complicated conditions. Internal tracheal stent placement with a silicone prosthesis was first attempted in
1965 by Montgomery. Since then, various stents have been used, including
those made of silicone and metal. The obvious advantages of stents are their
less invasive nature and the shorter surgical recovery times. However, complications include granulation tissue formation, difficult removal, stent frac-
ture, the need for additional stent placement, migration, the need to further
dilate the stent as the child grows, and death. An advantage of the silicone
stent is its relatively easy removal and the deployment of a larger stent, if
required, as the child grows. Metallic, self-expanding stents have been cata-
strophic in many cases. Removability is especially important because children stand a reasonable chance of becoming asymptomatic once the
airway grows. Currently, stents are used in limited situations in which conventional therapy has failed. However, stents currently in development, such
as resorbable biopolymer stents [17], may address the limitations of those in
current use.

Congenital tracheal stenosis and complete tracheal rings

Congenital tracheal stenosis (CTS) in neonates and infants is an under-
diagnosed, life-threatening, respiratory anomaly. The absence of the membranous portion of the trachea can create local or generalized stenosis
[18,19]. Backer and Mavroudis defined tracheal stenosis as a reduction in
the anatomic luminal diameter of the trachea by more than 50%, compared
with the remaining normal trachea [20,21]. Chen and Holinger have proposed
that the formation of complete or near-complete tracheal rings arises from
disproportionate growth of the cartilage relative to the posterior tracheal
pars membranacea [22]. In addition to near-complete tracheal rings, the infant may also be affected by a vertical fusion of the tracheal cartilage (tracheal cartilaginous sleeve). Furthermore, Voland and colleagues [23] have
proposed that an intrinsic field defect in the cervical splanchnic mesenchyme
may account for the presence of complete tracheal rings and the frequent association of mediastinal and cervical chondrogenic anomalies like a foreshortened neck and trachea, pulmonary agenesis, and abnormal vasculature.

The CTS has been classified into three principal types: (1) generalized hypoplasia, (2) funnel-like narrowing, and (3) segmental stenosis. The stenotic
segment is most often composed of completely circular "O" rings of cartilage. Alternatively, disorganized cartilages, ridges, or plates of cartilage
may occur (Fig. 5). Type I CTS is when all or most of the trachea is stenotic.
Type II CTS is a funnel stenosis, variously located and of variable length.

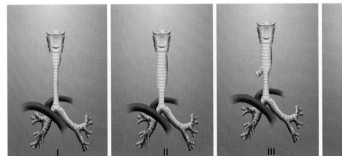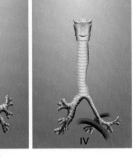

Fig. 5. Types of CTS. Type I: All or most of the trachea is stenosed. Type II: Funnel stenosis is variously located and of variable length. Type III: short, segmental stenosis, sometimes below an anomalous right upper lobe bronchus. Type IV: Anomalous right upper lobe bronchus with a 'bronchus' to horizontally branching bronchi to the rest of the lung. The right upper lobe bronchus is at the normal carinal level. The bridge bronchus is stenotic, and lesser stenosis may involve part of the trachea above. In some cases, the trachea is elongated as shown, but the upper lobe bronchus is absent. Location of the left pulmonary artery sling is indicated when present.

Type III CTS is a short, segmental stenosis, sometimes below an anomalous right upper lobe bronchus, and type IV CTS occurs when there is an anomalous right upper lobe bronchus with a 'bronchus' to horizontally branching bronchi to the rest of the lung. The right upper lobe bronchus is at the normal carinal level. The bridge bronchus is stenotic, and lesser stenosis may involve part of the trachea above. In more than one half of patients, CTS may be accompanied by other malformations, including cardiac and pulmonary anomalies, inguinal hernias, imperforate anus, radial aplasia, megaureters and other ureteral anomalies, Down syndrome, and Pfeiffer syndrome. Segmental stenosis of the distal trachea may be associated with an aberrant left pulmonary artery, the so-called "pulmonary artery sling" (Fig. 6) or "ring sling complex." The left pulmonary artery originates from the proximal portion of the right artery and passes behind the trachea to the left lung. In this course, it indents, but rarely obstructs, the esophagus. One must be aware of this anomaly when examining an infant with apparent segmental distal tracheal stenosis. The association between vascular slings and complete tracheal rings is so strong that the discovery of one of these anomalies is an indication to search actively for the other.

Symptoms are variable, depending on the age of the child, the degree of stenosis, and the potential presence of associated anomalies. Length of stenosis does not appear to be as critical as degree of stenosis in producing symptoms, because airway resistance is only linearly proportional to length of stenosis, whereas resistance increases fourfold relative to a decrease in the luminal diameter. These infants present with stridor, retractions, and increased work of breathing and dying spells. A characteristic clinical sign is the wet-sounding biphasic noise made by secretions being moved by airflow

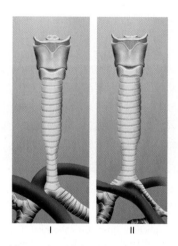

Fig. 6. Congenital stenosis with associated left pulmonary artery sling (the ring sling complex). (*I*) A short segment distal stenosis is present. (*II*) A bridge bronchus is adjacent to the anomalous artery. The apparent length of "trachea" is greater than that in *I*, and the bronchial branching approximates an inverted "T."

through an area of distal tracheal stenosis, termed "washing machine" breathing. A thorough bronchoscopic evaluation is required for the diagnosis. CT usually allows a correct diagnosis. If necessary, helical CT can be useful for evaluating dynamic changes in the airway. MRI is valuable for demonstrating the relationship of the airway to adjacent blood vessels without injection of intravascular contrast medium. CT and MRI can provide three-dimensional reconstruction.

Based on results reviewed in the literature, long-segment, funnel-shaped CTS should no longer be treated conservatively, except for very mild cases. Balloon dilatation has been partially successful, but a rupture of the tracheal wall that could lead to a mediastinitis is always associated with this procedure [24]. The management of complete tracheal rings remains controversial, as illustrated by the many surgical techniques advocated, including enlargement (using costal cartilage, pericardial patch, tracheal autograft) tracheoplasty, tracheal resection–anastomosis and slide tracheoplasty [25]. Rutter and colleagues [26], from the Cincinnati Children's Hospital, reported 11 cases of complete tracheal rings that had been treated by slide tracheoplasties with a cardiopulmonary bypass or an extracorporeal membrane oxygenation. They found this technique to be more efficient, with less morbidity and mortality. They made the important observation that although a trachea may improve with time after any type of tracheoplasty, it is uncommon for an adequately repaired trachea to deteriorate in the intermediate or long term. In their observation, the main factor associated with a poor outcome is a child who is severely compromised before tracheoplasty, especially with respect to nonairway pathologies.

Resection and reconstruction of the trachea

Resections and reconstruction of the trachea (Fig. 7) have been performed with considerable success in appropriate settings. Traditional concerns about avoiding anastomotic tension and the danger of postoperative obstruction due to edema and secretions remain valid. Technique, as ever, must be precise and meticulous. For anastomosis in children, it is preferable to use 5-0 interrupted polyglactin 910 (Vicryl) sutures because of their ease of handling and strength, and because they do not cause granulation tissue formation. In large numbers of cases, polyglactin 910 sutures are nearly ideal as tracheal anastomotic sutures in terms of ease of use, strength, minimal reactivity, and, most important, absence of long-term complications such a granulomas, suture erosion into the lumen, and anastomotic separation and stenosis. Polydioxanone monofilament suture is somewhat more difficult to handle and has no advantages.

Enlargement tracheoplasty

In 1982, Kimura and colleagues [27] described anterior patch tracheoplasty (see Fig. 7) for treatment of congenital stenosis involving the entire trachea. A stenosis too long to be treated by resection and anastomosis was incised vertically throughout its length, and the tracheal diameter was widened by fitting a long cartilage graft. An endotracheal tube was left in place until the patch became firm. Idriss and colleagues [28] modified the procedure by using pericardium, which required not only postoperative splinting with an endotracheal tube but suture suspension of the pliable pericardial patch to mediastinal structures. Considerable difficulty was encountered with granulation tissue formation, necessitating multiple postoperative bronchoscopies (mean 3.8), especially for grafts extending distally (mean

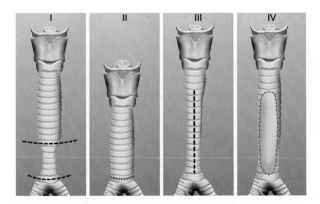

Fig. 7. Surgical treatment of CTS. (*I*) Resection and reconstruction, suitable only for shorter stenosis. (*II*) Patch tracheoplasty. Incision and tracheal widening with free cartilage or pericardial grafts.

complication rate 16) [28]. Twenty-one patients underwent pericardial patch repair, with two operative deaths and three late deaths [29]. Six needed later tracheostomy, and two required airway stenting. Jaquiss and colleagues [30] advocated cartilage patch tracheoplasty. Their surgeries were complicated by granulation and, in one of six, dehiscence, but all their patients survived. Mechanical ventilatory support was provided for a mean of 11 days, with a median postoperative hospitalization of 17 days. In time, cartilage grafts are also replaced by mature scar tissue and re-epithelized by ciliated columnar epithelium.

Slide tracheoplasty

Slide tracheoplasty (Figs. 8–11) can be performed under conventional anesthesia (intubation with a small-bore endotracheal tube). For shorter stenoses of the lower half of the trachea, an approach through a right thoracotomy also is possible. The anterior wall of the trachea is exposed and the stenosis measured, with the help of a simultaneous bronchoscopy when necessary. The trachea is then divided transversally, exactly at the midpoint of its narrowed segment. The proximal end is mobilized circumferentially and then divided longitudinally along its posterior wall, extending across all complete rings to the full length of the stricture. The distal segment is mobilized only partially, to preserve its vascularization. It also is divided longitudinally, but along its anterior border down to the length of the stenosis as far as the carina, or farther if necessary. The ends of both segments are spatulated and the two tracheal segments are approximated by sliding one over the other (hence, the term slide tracheoplasty), and sutured together with separated submucosal sutures. The circumference of the airway is doubled, the diameter shows a fourfold increase, and the trachea is shortened by exactly one half of the initial length of the stenosis, which is one half the shortening effect of resection and primary anastomosis. The

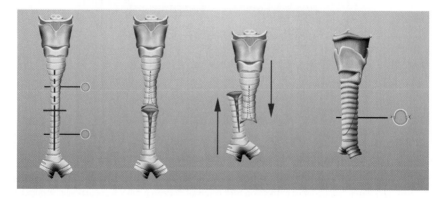

Fig. 8. Slide tracheoplasty.

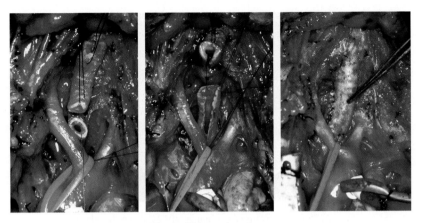

Fig. 9. Slide tracheoplasty.

excellent tracheal stability obtained by this technique allows early extubation [25]. The formation of inflammatory granulations in the tracheal lumen
is minimal postoperatively, because the whole endoluminal surface is covered by mucosa, and there is no mesenchymal graft. Despite the extensive
tracheal mobilization, particularly at the level of the superior segment, no
lesion of the recurrent nerves or problem of devascularization of the trachea
has been observed [25]. Careful preservation of the blood supply of the inferior tracheal segment seems sufficient to allow tissue healing.

Comparing the two techniques in terms of postoperative recovery and
midterm results, the duration of postoperative intubation is shorter after
a slide tracheoplasty (less than 24 hours), compared with mean values of
7 to 12 days (extreme values ranging from 6–48 days) after enlargement tracheoplasty. Endoluminal granulations present a minor problem after slide
tracheoplasty, requiring fewer endoscopic procedures compared with

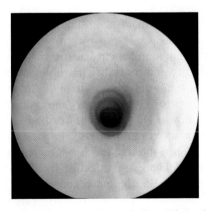

Fig. 10. Preoperative tracheal lumen (before slide tracheoplasty).

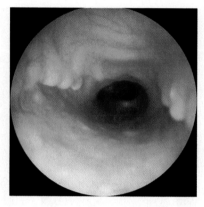

Fig. 11. Postoperative tracheal lumen (after slide tracheoplasty).

a mean of 13 such interventions after enlargement tracheoplasty (extreme values ranging from 3.8–16.8) [2,29,31] No open surgical revisions were needed in the slide tracheoplasty series, whereas a large number of enlargement tracheoplasties had to be reoperated (5 of 15 [32], 3 of 12 [2], 7 of 28 [33]), mainly because of luminal obstruction, graft rupture, or recurrence of the stenosis. A slide tracheoplasty resulted in no recurrent nerve injuries and no problem of tracheal devascularization [31,34–36]. Functional mid-term results of the slide tracheoplasty seem to be superior to those of enlargement tracheoplasty. None of the survivors of slide tracheoplasty have been recanulated or have shown respiratory limitations [25]. After enlargement tracheoplasty, 2 of 23 patients [29] had a long-term tracheostomy, and 60% of the patients [32] had persistent dyspnea [2] or needed a stent for adequate respiration. No long-term results are available for patients after slide tracheoplasty because the longest follow-up to evaluate tracheal growth has been 3.5 years [33]. However, because the trachea seems to grow well after an enlargement tracheoplasty, or resection and anastomosis, problems with tracheal growth after a slide tracheoplasty would not be expected [35].

Children with CTS and complex cardiac anomalies are thought to carry a higher risk of morbidity and mortality. Pathologic hemodynamics, in addition to obstructing a small-dimension airway with its known mucosal reactivity, leave little room for compensatory mechanisms, especially during respiratory tract infections [37]. When the cardiac lesion is repaired first, the patient usually has severe, and often fatal, respiratory trouble in the postoperative period. When the tracheal lesion is repaired first, the postoperative risk of wound dehiscence and infection increases because of impaired microcirculation, hypoxia, or both, and because of the tissue and malnutrition. It is therefore important to perform effective surgical relief of both disease entities concomitantly to obtain better operative results.

Healing of the juvenile trachea after tracheoplasty
or a resection-anastomosis: growth and tension

The question of whether anastomosis performed in the juvenile trachea will grow adequately has been answered. Maeda and Grillo [38] demonstrated experimentally that tracheal anastomosis in puppies resulted in more narrowing at the anastomotic site than in adult dogs. It is caused by the infolding of adjacent rings and the restriction of growth by scarring of the membranous wall. At the anastomotic site, the average growth was 82% of normal sagittally, and 75% coronally, values equivalent to 20% stenosis of the tracheal lumen. Tension on the anastomosis caused by resection of progressively longer segments of trachea led to greater anastomotic narrowing when performed in puppies than in adult animals.

As experience with tracheal resection and reconstruction in infants and children increased, clinical results confirmed these expectations of anastomotic growth. Couraud and colleagues [39] observed growth following similar laryngotracheal procedures. Intolerance of anastomotic tension in the juvenile trachea confirmed the desirability of confining resection in children to 25% to 30% of the tracheal length.

Growth of tracheal cartilage appears to occur continuously on the convex or outer side of a ring, with resorption taking place on the concave side, without identifiable growth centers. Serial bronchoscopic observations of unoperated congenital stenoses have shown that the stenotic segment grows in proportion to the normal trachea. Manson and colleagues [40] demonstrated this growth radiologically. Macchiarini and colleagues [41] observed growth in an experimental model approximating slide tracheoplasty for long congenital stenosis. Such growth has now been confirmed clinically by Grillo and colleagues [38,42].

Laryngotracheal clefts

Congenital laryngeal clefts (LCs) and (LTECs) occur in approximately 1 of 2000 live births. According to Benjamin and Inglis [43], four types can be distinguished: type I is a supraglottic arytenoid cleft; type II is a partial cricoid cleft extending beyond the level of the vocal cords; type III is a total cricoid cleft extending into the cervical trachea; and type IV is an LTEC extending into the thoracic trachea and, occasionally, into one or both main bronchi. Neonates present with a hoarse cry, the inability to handle secretions, cyanosis, choking, coughing, stridor, and recurrent pneumonia, depending on the length of the cleft. Because laryngotracheal clefts are very rare congenital anomalies, no single institution has sufficient experience to propose a general algorithm for treatment. Furthermore, different investigators suggest different classifications. The potential association of clefts with other congenital anomalies clouds the evaluation outcome measures after surgery. The international pediatric community badly needs a consensus conference on a universally accepted classification, if one wishes to compare results with different treatment modalities. For instance, in some articles a type III cleft reaches the intrathoracic trachea down to the carina, whereas in others, this same type corresponds to a complete posterior cricoid cleft only [44]. Taking into consideration the above-mentioned drawbacks and the need for a more accurate distinction among the different extents of LTECs, the authors' institution has used a modified Benjamin's classification (Fig. 12). It has the advantage of providing a clear distinction among partial cricoid clefts (type II), total cricoid clefts (type IIIa), and extrathoracic LTECs extending down to the level of the sternal notch (type IIIb), but not involving the intrathoracic trachea. To compare the success rates of cleft repairs extending down to the sternal notch, notably with open or endoscopic approaches, this classification is necessary. For type I and some minor type II clefts, endoscopic repair is the preferred option. Myer and colleagues [45] recommended surgical management of types II, IIIa and b, and IVa and b LTECs by an anterior laryngofissure or lateral pharyngotomy, with an option to perform a thoracotomy for distal access. In advanced LTECs, the lateral pharyngotomy provides visualization of both the tracheal and esophageal defects with a relatively easy access to the entire length of the defect. Thus, lateral pharyngotomy is the approach of choice for complete LTECs. Critics of open approaches are concerned about destabilization of an already deficient larynx, though this worry has not been supported in animal studies. External approaches also place the recurrent laryngeal nerves at increased risk of injury [46]. Some investigators have advocated interposing vascularized tissue such as sternocleidomastoid or pectoralis muscle, parietal pleura, or a tibia periosteal graft to reinforce the closure [44].

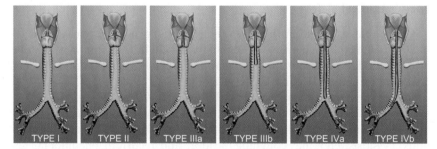

Fig. 12. Classification of Laryngotracheal clefts. Type 0: Submucosal cleft. Type I: Interarytenoid cleft with absence of the interarytenoid muscle. Type II: Posterior cleft extending partially through the cricoid plate. Type IIIa: Posterior cleft extending down to the inferior border of the cricoid plate. Type IIIb: Posterior cleft extending into the cervical trachea, but not further down than the level of the sternal notch. Type IVa: Laryngotracheal cleft extending into the intrathoracic trachea to the carina. Type IVb: Intrathoracic extension of the cleft involving one main bronchus.

Using modern technology with fine carbon dioxide–laser incisions and endoscopic suturing (Figs. 13 and 14), the authors' experience shows that endoscopic repair of type I through IIIb clefts is now possible, without intubation or tracheotomy (Figs. 15–17). The only prerequisite for this endoscopic approach is the absence of other airway anomalies (laryngomalacia, tracheomalacia, TEF) and of associated congenital anomalies (Pallister-Hall and Opitz-Frias syndromes), which may require creation of a safe airway with intubation or tracheotomy. The endoscopic approach offers several advantages over conventional open surgeries. An anterior incision of the larynx and trachea is avoided, as is the need for postoperative intubation or tracheotomy, which diminishes the potential risk of destabilizing the laryngotracheal framework and avoids the increased risk of wound breakdown related to the nasotracheal tube or the tracheotomy cannula. Furthermore, by repairing the cleft through the endoscopic route, the surgeon has a constant axial view of the airway that needs to be reconstructed. It is thus easy to avoid the inclusion of excess mucosa into the reconstructed airway, which potentially would lead to laryngotracheal stenosis. Additionally, this minimally invasive technique preserves the vascular supply to the mucosa used for the repair, and the presence of redundant mucosa in the postcricoid and esophageal regions allows a tight closure of the second mucosal layer. This result is much more difficult to achieve through the open translaryngotracheal approach. Finally, the risk of recurrent laryngeal nerve injury is nil. In the postoperative period, no tracheal intubation or tracheotomy is necessary. Usually, the laryngeal edema induced by the cleft repair is minimal, and CPAP or biphasic positive airway pressure helps prevent airway collapse during the inspiratory phase of respiration.

The repair technique for complete LTECs is only one aspect of the management of these patients. Before repair, the airway is often difficult to

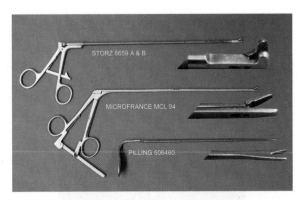

Fig. 13. Instruments used for endoscopic suturing. Karl Storz (8659 A & B for right and left) and Microfrance (MCL 94) needle-holders allow the small "TF plus" needle used for suturing to be grasped firmly. A Pilling pusher (506480) is used for tying the knots.

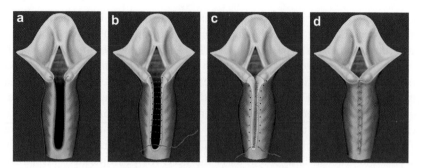

Fig. 14. The principle of endoscopic laryngotracheal cleft repair. (*a*) With the CO_2 laser in the ultrapulse mode (150 mJ/cm2, 10 Hz), a sharp incision at the mucosal border of the cleft is made (*red line*). (*b*) The first inner layer of suturing is done on the tracheal side, with the knots tied on the pharyngoesophageal side of the repair. (*c*) The second layer of suturing uses the redundant mucosa of the esophagus and pharynx to get a tight closure on the pharyngoesophageal side of the repair. (*d*) Completion of the endoscopic repair. No knots are visible in the trachea because they are all tied on the pharyngeal side of the repair; the first row of stitches is buried in the wound by the second mucosal layer.

maintain. Often, tracheotomy is suggested; however, with some severe deformities, a tracheotomy may not secure the airway adequately. Custom-made, bifurcated endotracheal and tracheotomy tubes have been described for maintaining these difficult airways with reasonable success. Gastric reflux is a common finding in patients who have LCs or LTECs. The unprotected airway is exposed to the gastric contents, resulting in an inflamed bronchopulmonary tree and aspiration pneumonia. The common surgical procedures for gastric reflux include Nissen fundoplication or a Roux-en-Y gastrojejunostomy, truncal vagotomy, and partial fundoplication. In addition to needing surgical management of the reflux, these patients require

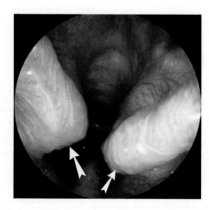

Fig. 15. Preoperative endoscopic view of a type IIIb cleft repair. The distal end of the cleft lies much lower than the inferior border of the cricoid plate (*white arrows*).

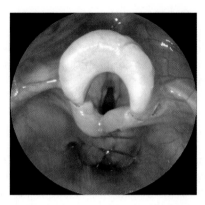

Fig. 16. Immediate postoperative endoscopic view at completion of the cleft repair. Only the two uppermost stitches of the seven rows of sutures are visible.

aggressive antireflux protocols at the time of diagnosis, including medical management with proton pump inhibitors, prokinetic agents, or histamine-2 antagonists; reverse Trendelenburg positioning; and proximal gastric drainage.

Nutritional status is another significant aspect to the preoperative and postoperative care of those patients who have complete airway clefts. These infants must have sufficient caloric and protein intake to meet the metabolic demands associated with wound healing and neonatal growth. The time from diagnosis to reconstruction should be as short as possible to decrease the degree of reflux-induced esophagotracheitis and pulmonary aspiration.

Outcome has improved since the 1950s. Survival for LC or LTEC repair has improved from 18% in the period from 1955 to 1970, to 75% in 1984. In their review of 85 patients in 1983, Roth and colleagues [47] found a 43%

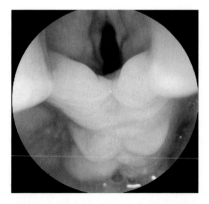

Fig. 17. Postoperative result at 6 months. The cleft repair is healed fully without recurrent fistula. The interarytenoid space is estimated at about 50% of the normal distance in the fully abducted position of the vocal cords.

mortality with types I and II LCs, 42% mortality with type III LTECs, and 93% mortality with type IV LTECs [44]. In the authors' reported four cases of type IIIa and b clefts that were treated by endoscopic means only, all infants could resume spontaneous respiration without support, and normal feeding, within an average of less than 12 days.

Other anomalies

Tracheal bronchus was described by Sandifort in 1785 as a right upper bronchus originating in the trachea. The term tracheal bronchus includes various bronchial anomalies arising in the trachea or main bronchus and directed toward the upper lobe territory. This anomalous bronchus usually exits the right lateral wall of the trachea less than 2 cm above the major carina, and can supply the entire upper lobe or its apical segment. A tracheal bronchus may be displaced or may be supernumerary. Right tracheal bronchus has a prevalence of 0.1% to 2%, and left tracheal bronchus a prevalence of 0.3% to 1%, in bronchographic and bronchoscopic studies. Patients are usually asymptomatic, but the diagnosis of tracheal bronchus should be considered in cases of persistent or recurrent upper lobe pneumonia, atelectasis or air trapping, and chronic bronchitis. Bronchiectasis, focal emphysema, and cystic lung malformations may coexist. Most of these bronchial branching anomalies are well-diagnosed on chest CT as small areas of hypoattenuation arising directly from the trachea. Most patients who have tracheal bronchus do not require treatment; however, in symptomatic patients, surgical excision of the involved segment may be necessary.

Congenital fistula between biliary and respiratory tracts is extraordinarily rare [12]. Respiratory problems begin with cough and progress to intractable pneumonia. The most common location of the fistula is at the carina, but right and left bronchial connections have been noted. Yellow fluid is identified bronchoscopically. Contrast will identify a long paraesophageal tract connecting to a hepatic duct. This condition has also been seen in a young adult [12]. Excision of the intrathoracic segment with closure at the carina (or bronchus) and at the diaphragmatic level cures this problem.

Tracheal webs sometime occur in the neonatal and juvenile trachea at the cricoid level, though laryngeal webs at the glottic level are more common. Tracheal webs are usually short and are generally treated endoscopically by laser or a short tracheal resection with end-to-end anastomosis.

Tracheobronchomegaly (Mounier-Kuhn disease) appears to be of congenital origin, but most patients do not become significantly symptomatic until midlife. In hindsight, symptoms can often be traced back to youth. The condition is very rare and is thought to be caused by the absence of the trachealis muscle. The anterior tracheal wall may become indented as the rings fold backward.

Congenital high airway obstruction syndrome and the ex utero intrapartum treatment procedure

The prenatal sonographic findings of bilateral, uniformly enlarged echogenic lungs, flattened or inverted diaphragms, dilated airways, and mediastinal compression are indicative of complete, or nearly complete, obstruction of the upper fetal airway. When these findings are associated with fetal hydrops, a diagnosis of congenital high airway obstruction syndrome (CHAOS) is made [48,49]. This condition can be caused by tracheal agenesis or atresia, or large laryngotracheal cysts [9]. The ex utero intrapartum treatment (EXIT) procedure allows time for an airway to be established in a careful, controlled manner before delivery, while uteroplacental gas exchange is preserved. In addition, the consequences of tracheal obstruction including capillary leak syndrome, respiratory distress syndrome, tracheobronchial malacia, and diaphragmatic dysfunction are all reversible and tracheal reconstruction is feasible. Maternal laparotomy and hysterotomy is performed under deep inhalational anesthesia to ensure uterine relaxation and to preserve uteroplacental gas exchange. While on placental support, the fetal head and neck are exposed and a laryngotracheoscopy is performed. A fetal tracheostomy is performed, surfactant is administered by way of a tracheostomy, and ventilation is established before clamping and dividing the umbilical cord. The infant may suffer from severe respiratory distress syndrome initially, but generally responds to surfactant therapy. This approach allows time to evaluate and treat the underlying pathology. It is uncertain what effect fetal tracheotomy has on lung development in fetuses with CHAOS. In experimental animal models, chronic drainage of tracheal fluid, as would occur with fetal tracheotomy, results in pulmonary hypoplasia. In the past, the fetus with airway compromise due to CHAOS has been at high risk for anoxic brain injury or death after conventional cesarean section or vaginal delivery because of the long time required to secure the newborn airway. Application of the EXIT procedure in cases of CHAOS offers the potential for salvage and excellent long-term outcome.

References

[1] Willliams PL, Warwick R, editors. Gray's anatomy. 36th edition. Philadelphia: WB Saunders; 1980. p. 1246.

[2] Bando K, Turrentine MW, Sun K, et al. Anterior pericardial tracheoplasty for congenital tracheal stenosis: intermediate to long-term outcomes. Ann Thorac Surg 1996;62:981–9.

[3] Das BB, Nagaraj A, Rao HA, et al. Tracheal agenesis: report of three cases and review of literature. Am J Perinatol 2002;19:395–9.

[4] Floyd J, Campbell DC, Domini DE. Agenesis of the trachea. Am Rev Respir Dis 1962;86: 557–60 [no abstract available].

[5] Kluth D, Steding G, Seidl W. The embryology of foregut malformations. J Pediatr Surg 1987;22:389–93.

[6] Baarsma R, Bekedam DJ, Visser GHA. Qualitative abnormal fetal breathing movements, associated with tracheal atresia. Early Hum Dev 1993;32:63–9.

[7] Grillo HC. Surgery of the trachea and bronchi. Hamilton (Canada): BC Decker Inc.; 2004.

[8] Diaz EM, Adams JM, Hawkins HK, et al. Tracheal agenesis. Arch Otolaryngol Head Neck Surg 1989;115:741–5.

[9] Crombleholme TM, Sylvester K, Alan W, et al. Salvage of a fetus with congenital high airway obstruction syndrome by ex utero intrapartum treatment (EXIT) procedure. Fetal Diagn Ther 2000;15:280–2.

[10] Benjamin B. Tracheomalacia in infants and children. Ann Otol Rhinol Laryngol 1984;93:438–42.

[11] Grillo HC, Zannini P. Management of obstructive tracheal disease in children. J Pediatr Surg 1984;19:414–6.

[12] An update on the pediatric airway. Otolaryngol Clin North Am 2000.

[13] Jacobs IN, Wetmore RF, Tom LW, et al. Tracheobronchomalacia in children. Arch Otolaryngol Head Neck Surg 1994;120:154–8.

[14] Kelly A Carden, Philip M Boiselle, David A Waltz, et-al. Tracheomalacia and tracheobronchomalacia in children and adults: an in-depth review. Chest 2005;127:984–1005.

[15] Bullard KM, Scott Adzick N, Harrison MR. A mediastinal window approach to aortopexy. J Pediatr Surg 1997;32:680–1.

[16] Hagl S, Jakob H, Sebening C, et al. External stabilization of long-segment tracheobronchomalacia guided by intraoperative bronchoscopy. Ann Thorac Surg 1997;64(5):1412–21.

[17] Sewall GK, Warner T, Conner NP, et al. Comparison of resorbable poly-L-lactic acid-polyglycolic acid and internal Palmaz stents for the surgical correction of severe tracheomalacia. Ann Otol Rhinol Laryngol 2003;112:515–21.

[18] Grillo HC, Wright CD, Vlahakes GJ, et al. Management of congenital tracheal stenosis by means of slide tracheoplasty or resection and reconstruction, with long-term follow-up of growth after slide tracheoplasty. J Thorac Cardiovasc Surg 2002;123:145–52.

[19] Dodge-Khatami A, Tsang VT, Roebuck DJ, et al. Management of congenital tracheal stenosis: a multidisciplinary approach. Images Paediatr Cardiol 2000;2:29–39.

[20] Wright CD, Graham BB, Eng M, et al. Paediatric tracheal surgery. Ann Thorac Surg 2002;74:308–14.

[21] Backer CL, Mavroudis C. Congenital heart surgery nomenclature and database project: vascular rings, tracheal stenosis, pectus excavatum. Ann Thorac Surg 2000;69(Suppl):S308–18.

[22] Chen JC, Holinger LD. Congenital tracheal anomalies: pathology study using serial macrosections and review of the literature. Pediatr Pathol 1994;14:513–37.

[23] Voland JR, Benirschke K, Saunders B. Congenital tracheal stenosis with associated cardiopulmonary anomalies. Pediatr Pulmonol 1986;2:247–9.

[24] Messineo A, Forte V, Joseph T, et al. The balloon posterior tracheal split: a technique for managing tracheal stenosis in the premature infant. J Pediatr Surg 1992;27:1142–4.

[25] Lang FJ, Hurni M, Monnier P. Long segment congenital tracheal stenosis: treatment by slide-tracheoplasty. J Pediatr Surg 1999;34:1216–22.

[26] Rutter MJ, Cotton RT, Azizkhan RG, et al. Slide tracheoplasty for the management of complete tracheal ring. J Pediatr Surg 2003;38(6):928–34.

[27] Kimura K, Mukohara N, Tsugawa C, et al. Tracheoplasty for congenital stenosis of the entire trachea. J Pediatr Surg 1982;17:869–71.

[28] Idriss FS, DeLeon SY, Ilbawi MS, et al. Tracheoplasty with pericardial patch for extensive tracheal stenosis in infants and children. J Thorac Cardiovasc Surg 1984;88:527–36.

[29] Dunham ME, Holinger LD, Backer CL, et al. Management of severe congenital tracheal stenosis. Ann Otol Rhinol Laryngol 1994;103:351–6.

[30] Jaquiss RDB, Lusk PR, Spray TL, et al. Repair of long-segment tracheal stenosis in infancy. J Thorac Cadiovasc Surg 1995;110:1504–12.

[31] Dayan SH, Dunham ME, Backer CL, et al. Slide-tracheoplasty in the management of congenital tracheal stenosis. Ann Otol Rhinol Laryngol 1997;106:914–9.

[32] Andrews TM, Cotton RT, Bailey WW, et al. Tracheoplasty for congenital complete tracheal rings. Arch Otolaryngol Head Neck Surg 1994;120:1363–9.

[33] Backer CL, Maroudis C, Dunham ME, et al. Reoperation after pericardial patch tracheoplasty. J Pediatr Surg 1997;32:1108–12.

[34] Tsang V, Murday A, Gilbe C, et al. Slide tracheoplasty for congenital funnel-shaped stenosis. Ann Thorac Surg 1989;48:632–5.

[35] Grillo HC. Slide-tracheoplasty for long-segment congenital tracheal stenosis. Ann Thorac Surg 1994;58:613–21.

[36] Tsang V, Goldstraw P. Tracheal approach to pulmonary artery sling associated with funnel-shaped tracheal stenosis. Cardiovasc Surg 1993;1:300–2.

[37] Loukanov T, Sebening C, Springer W, et al. Simultaneous management of congenital tracheal stenosis and cardiac anomalies in infants. J Thorac Cardiovasc Surg 2005;130(6): 1537–41.

[38] Maeda M, Grillo HC. Effect of tension on tracheal growth after resection and anastomosis in puppies. J Thorac Cardiovasc Surg 1973;65:658–68.

[39] Couraud L, Moreau JM, Velly JF. The growth of circumferential scars of the major airways from infancy to adulthood. Eur J Cardiothorac Surg 1990;4:521–6.

[40] Manson D, Filler R, Gordon R. Tracheal growth in congenital tracheal stenosis. Pediatr Radiol 1996;26:427–30.

[41] Macchiari P, Sulmet E, de Montpreville V, et al. Tracheal growth after slide tracheoplasty. J Thorac Cardiovasc Surg 1997;113:558–66.

[42] Grillo HC, Wright CD, Vlahakes GJ, et al. Management of congenital tracheal stenosis by means of tracheoplasty or resection and reconstruction, with long term follow-up of growth after slide tracheoplasty. J Thorac Cadiovasc Surg 1994;107:600–6.

[43] Benjamin B, Inglis A. Minor congenital laryngeal clefts: diagnosis and classification. Ann Otol Rhinol Laryngol 1989;98:417–20.

[44] Sandu K, Monnier P. Endoscopic laryngotracheal cleft repair without tracheotomy or intubation. Laryngoscope 2006;116:630–4.

[45] Myer CM, Cotton RT, Holmes DK, et al. Laryngeal and laryngotracheoesophageal clefts: role of early surgical repair. Ann Otol Rhinol Laryngol 1990;99:98–104.

[46] Garabedian EN, Ducroz V, Roger G, et al. Posterior laryngeal clefts: preliminary report of a new surgical procedure using tibial periosteum as an interposition graft. Laryngoscope 1998;108:899–902.

[47] Roth B, Rose K-G, Benz-Bohm G, et al. Laryngotracheo-oesophageal cleft. Clinical features, diagnosis and therapy. Eur J Paediatr 1983;140:41–6.

[48] Hedrick MH, Ferro MM, Filly RA, et al. Congenital high airway obstruction syndrome (CHAOS): a potential for perinatal intervention. J Pediatr Surg 1992;29:272–4.

[49] Berrocal T, Madrid C, Novo S, et al. Congenital anomalies of the tracheobronchial tree, lung, and mediastinum: embryology, radiology, and pathology. Radiographics 2004;24:e17.

ELSEVIER
SAUNDERS

Otolaryngol Clin N Am
40 (2007) 219–244

OTOLARYNGOLOGIC
CLINICS
OF NORTH AMERICA

Congenital Anomalies of the Esophagus

Olga Achildi, BA[a],
Harsh Grewal, MD, FACS, FAAP[a,b],*

[a]*Department of Surgery, Temple University School of Medicine,
3420 North Broad Street, Philadelphia, PA 19140, USA*
[b]*Section of Pediatric Surgery, Department of Surgery, Temple University Children's
Medical Center, 3509 North Broad Street, 5 East, Philadelphia, PA 19140, USA*

Normal anatomy and embryology of the esophagus

The esophagus is a hollow muscular tube consisting of mucosa, submucosa, and muscularis layers. The mucosa is composed of stratified squamous nonkeratinized epithelium that transitions to columnar epithelium at the gastroesophageal junction. The esophagus lacks a serosal layer. The muscle layer consists of striated muscle in the upper one third and smooth muscle in the lower two thirds of the tube; these are arranged as an inner circular and an outer longitudinal layer (Fig. 1). During ingestion of a meal, distention of the proximal striated muscle initiates peristalsis, which continues down the esophagus and is coordinated by the medullary centers (nucleus ambiguus and dorsal motor nucleus) and the vagus nerve (Fig. 2). The Auerbach's (myenteric) plexus is found between the circular and longitudinal muscles and mediates intrinsic motor control of the esophagus, whereas the Meissner's plexus is located within the submucosa and innervates the lamina muscularis mucosae; these are part of the parasympathetic nervous system.

Two sphincters control passage of contents into the gastrointestinal tract: an anatomic upper esophageal sphincter (UES) and a physiologic lower esophageal sphincter (LES). The UES consists of cricopharyngeus and inferior pharyngeal constrictors, whereas the LES is histologically indistinguishable from the smooth muscle fibers of the lower esophagus.

Blood supply of the esophagus is segmental and is dictated by its anatomic location: the cervical portion receives blood supply from branches of the inferior thyroid artery, the thoracic portion from bronchial arteries and direct

---

* Corresponding author. Section of Pediatric Surgery, Department of Surgery, Temple University Children's Medical Center, 3509 North Broad Street, 5 East, Philadelphia, PA 19140.

E-mail address: harsh.grewal@temple.edu (H. Grewal).

0030-6665/07/$ - see front matter © 2007 Elsevier Inc. All rights reserved.
doi:10.1016/j.otc.2006.10.010   *oto.theclinics.com*

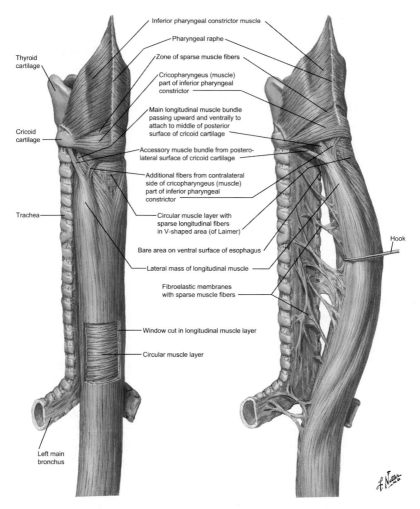

Thyroid cartilage

Cricoid cartilage

Trachea

Left main bronchus

Inferior pharyngeal constrictor muscle

Pharyngeal raphe

Zone of sparse muscle fibers

Cricopharyngeus (muscle) part of inferior pharyngeal constrictor

Main longitudinal muscle bundle passing upward and ventrally to attach to middle of posterior surface of cricoid cartilage

Accessory muscle bundle from postero-lateral surface of cricoid cartilage

Additional fibers from contralateral side of cricopharyngeus (muscle) part of inferior pharyngeal constrictor

Circular muscle layer with sparse longitudinal fibers in V-shaped area (of Laimer)

Bare area on ventral surface of esophagus

Lateral mass of longitudinal muscle

Fibroelastic membranes with sparse muscle fibers

Window cut in longitudinal muscle layer

Circular muscle layer

Hook

Fig. 1. Musculature of esophagus. (Netter image reprinted with permission from Elsevier, Inc.)

branches from the aorta, and the abdominal portion from the left gastric and the inferior phrenic arteries (Fig. 3). Venous drainage from the submucosal ve-nous plexus follows the arterial supply in the cervical and abdominal portions, whereas the thoracic esophagus drains into the azygous and hemiazygous sys-tem (Fig. 4). Likewise, the lymphatic drainage of the esophagus is segmental, with the cervical portion draining into deep cervical lymph nodes, the thoracic portion into the superior and posterior mediastinal lymph nodes, and the ab-dominal portion into the gastric and celiac lymph nodes.

The embryogenesis of esophageal atresia (EA) and tracheoesophageal fis-tulae is not completely understood. During fetal development, the foregut is formed around the 20th day of gestation. On day 22, the pharyngeal groove

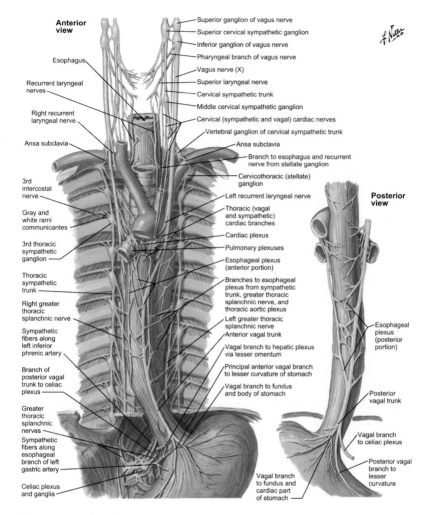

Fig. 2. Nerves of esophagus. (Netter image reprinted with permission from Elsevier, Inc.)

appears in the ventral aspect of the primitive foregut and within the next few days the lung bud forms at this locus. The mesenchyme between the foregut and the developing bronchial tree gives rise to the tracheoesophageal septum, and its proper development is believed to be necessary for the normal separation of the digestive and respiratory systems (Fig. 5).

The classic theory of division of respiratory and digestive tracts proposes that the tracheoesophageal septum forms as a pair of lateral folds that fuse in the midline to divide the esophagus from the trachea; this theory assumes that the lung buds develop from the trachea. More recent theories propose the development of paired symmetric diverticula from the primitive foregut in the absence of evidence for lateral folds forming a tracheoesophageal septum [1].

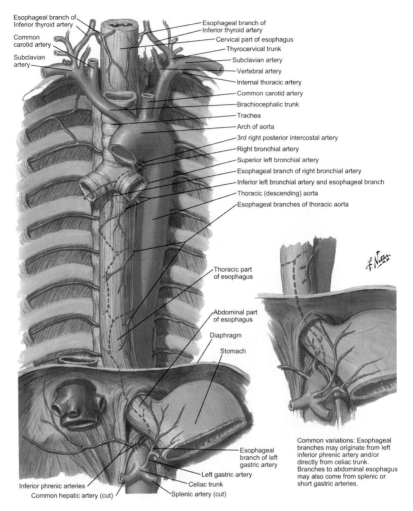

Fig. 3. Arteries of esophagus. (Netter image reprinted with permission from Elsevier, Inc.)

Esophageal atresia and tracheoesophageal fistula

History

EA was first reported by William Durston in 1670, and in 1697 Thomas Gibson described EA with tracheoesophageal fistula (TEF). The management of such malformations proved to be challenging, with the first unsuccessful attempt at TEF ligation in 1913 by Harry Richter who performed a transpleural ligation of the fistula and a gastrostomy to provide nutrition. From 1936 to 1938 Thomas Lanman and Robert Shaw independently attempted extrapleural ligations of TEF with primary anastomoses in five separate cases, all resulting in eventual death in the immediate postoperative

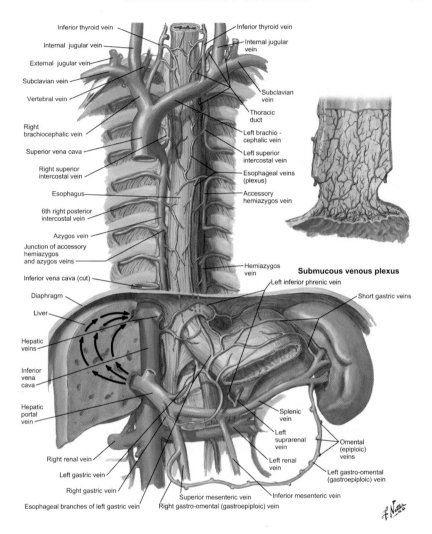

Fig. 4. Veins of esophagus. (Netter image reprinted with permission from Elsevier, Inc.)

period. The first survivors were reported independently by N. Logan Leven and William Ladd in 1939 using a multistaged approach that included placement of a gastrostomy tube, extrapleural division of TEF, and cervical esophagostomy. Gastrointestinal continuity was established using an antethoracic skin tube from the gastrostomy to esophagostomy. Although continuity was established, the repaired esophagus did not have normal peristalsis [2–4].

In 1941 Cameron Haight performed the first successful primary repair of EA with TEF after initial resuscitation of his 12-day-old patient by ligating the TEF using a left extrapleural approach followed by end-to-end

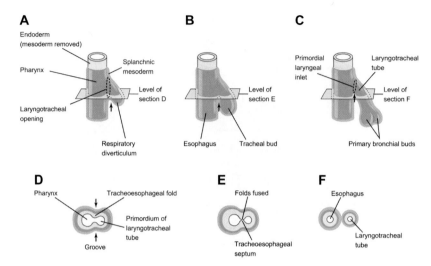

Fig. 5. Successive stages of development of the tracheoesophageal septum during the fourth and fifth weeks of development. (*A–C*) Lateral views of the caudal part of the primordial pharynx showing respiratory diverticulum and partitioning of the foregut into the esophagus and laryngotracheal tube. (*D–F*) Transverse sections illustrating formation of the tracheoesophageal septum and how it separates the foregut into the laryngotracheal tube and esophagus. (*From* The respiratory system. In: Moore KL, Persaud TVN, editors. Before we are born. Essentials of embryology and birth defects. 6th edition. Philadelphia: Saunders; 2003. p. 192; with permission.)

single layer anastomosis with interrupted silk sutures [4]. The operative treatment today still uses concepts used by these pioneering surgeons, with the biggest advancements being made in the supportive management of the postoperative neonate. The rates of survival have significantly improved from approximately 50% in the 1940s to greater than 90% today [2,3].

Classification

Initial classification system for EA was developed by E.C. Vogt in 1929. This system was slightly modified and the numerical nomenclature was transformed into an alphabetic one by Gross. This classification system groups the anomalies into: EA without TEF (type A), EA with proximal TEF (type B), EA with distal TEF (type C), EA with TEF between both esophageal segments and trachea (type D), TEF without EA or H-type fistula (type E), and esophageal stenosis (type F) (Fig. 6). Another classification system developed by Waterston and colleagues [5] in 1962 focused on risk factors and predicted survival in infants who have EA (Table 1). In the 1990s, Spitz and colleagues [6] included birth weight and presence of cardiac anomalies and proposed a system that is currently used as an alternative to the Waterston classification (Table 2).

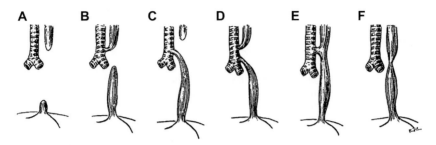

Fig. 6. Classification of congenital anomalies of the esophagus according to Gross. EA without TEF (*A*); EA with proximal TEF (*B*); EA with distal TEF (*C*); EA with TEF between both esophageal segments and trachea (*D*); TEF without EA or H-type fistula (*E*); and esophageal stenosis (*F*). (*From* Gross RE. Atresia of the esophagus. In: The surgery of infancy and childhood. Philadelphia: WB Saunders; 1953. p. 76; with permission.)

Epidemiology

The incidence of EA with or without TEF is approximately 2 in 10,000 births with a slight male predominance. Whites tend to be affected more often than non-whites. Increased incidence is seen in first pregnancies and advanced maternal age; the rate of chromosomal abnormalities and rate of twin pregnancy is increased from rates in the general population [2].

The most common anomaly is EA with distal TEF (Type C, 85%–90%), followed by EA alone (Type A, 7%–8%), TEF without EA (Type E, 4%–5%), EA with proximal TEF (Type B, ~1%), and EA with fistula to both pouches (Type E, ~1%) [2,3]. Associated congenital malformations are seen in approximately 50% of the cases; other gastrointestinal malformations are seen in 25% of the cases, and VACTERL association (vertebral/vascular, anorectal, cardiac, tracheoesophageal, radial/renal, limb deformities) occur in 20% of patients who have EA (Table 3) [7].

Embryogenesis of esophageal atresia

According to the classic theory, aberrant formation of the tracheoesophageal septum results from abnormal fusion of the lateral folds and may

Table 1
Waterston classification of esophageal atresia based on birth weight, presence of risk factors, and predicted survival

Group	Birth weight	General health	Survival
A	>2500 g	Otherwise healthy	100%
B	2000–2500 g	Otherwise healthy	85%
	>2500 g	Moderate associated anomalies (noncardiac, PDA, VSD, ASD)	
C	<2000 g	Otherwise healthy	65%
	>2000 g	Severe associated cardiac anomalies	

Abbreviations: ASD, atrial septal defect; PDA, patent ductus arteriosus; VSD, ventricular septal defect.

Table 2
Spitz classification of esophageal atresia based on birth weight, presence of cardiac defects, and predicted survival

Group	Characteristics	Survival rate
I	Birth wt > 1500 g, no major cardiac defects	97%
II	Birth wt < 1500 g or major cardiac defects	59%
III	Birth wt < 1500 g, major cardiac defects	22%

result in anomalous connections between the respiratory and digestive tracts. While studying chick embryos, however, Kluth and Fiegel [1] found no evidence of lateral folds during embryogenesis, but depicted a series of cranial and caudal folds in the region of tracheoesophageal separation. According to the chick embryo model, failure of appropriate development of these folds results in EA or tracheoesophageal fistula. Other investigators further demonstrated the role of epithelial proliferation and apoptosis in the development of the tracheoesophageal septum using the Adriamycin rat model [8,9].

Significant association of EA/TEF with other congenital anomalies implies a genetic link and has encouraged a search for possible responsible genes or chromosomal abnormalities. In various animal models tracheoesophageal malformations have been associated with mutations in the retinoic acid receptor (*RAR*), retinoid X receptor (*RXR*), sonic hedgehog (*shh*), thyroid transcription factor 1 (*TTF-1*), Gli family of zinc-finger transcription factors (*Gli1, Gli2, Gli3*), forkhead transcription factor (*Foxf1*), homeobox c4 (*Hoxc4*), and T-box transcription factor (*Tbx4*) [10]. The aberrant development of the digestive and respiratory tracts may be multifactorial and may involve numerous genetic and environmental factors that have yet to be elucidated.

Diagnosis

Prenatal diagnosis can be established by the presence of polyhydramnios, prominent esophageal pouch, and small or absent stomach "bubble" with fluid-filled loops of bowel on ultrasonography, usually in the third trimester of pregnancy. Polyhydramnios results from the inability of amniotic fluid to

Table 3
Incidence of other anomalies in patients who have esophageal atresia

Anomaly	Incidence
Cardiovascular	35%
Gastrointestinal	25%
Neurologic	25%
Musculoskeletal	20%
Renal	50%
VACTERL association	20%
Overall incidence	50%

reach the stomach in pure EA and decreased amniotic fluid ingestion in cases of TEF with or without EA. The positive predictive value of both polyhydramnios and a small or absent stomach is only 56%. Additional finding of the upper neck pouch sign, which is visualized during fetal swallowing, has high specificity for EA but may need a highly experienced operator [11].

Symptoms suspicious for EA/TEF can be observed shortly after birth and may include: excessive salivation; regurgitation, coughing, and choking following initial attempts to feed the neonate; respiratory distress; cyanosis; or inability to advance a catheter into the stomach. The nasogastric tube may curl in the proximal pouch suggesting atresia (Fig. 7). A distended, air-filled abdomen is suggestive of EA with a distal TEF (Type C) because of the passage of air from the trachea into the gastrointestinal tract. Findings on chest and abdominal radiograph include an air-filled blind pouch with EA, presence of air in the gastrointestinal tract in cases of distal TEF, and pneumonia because of the presence of gastric reflux into the lung from a distal TEF. If there is difficulty in making a diagnosis, a small quantity of nonionic water-soluble contrast or diluted barium can help outline the proximal pouch (Fig. 8). The presence of a proximal air-filled pouch and a gasless abdomen is suggestive of EA without TEF (Type A). Diagnosis of H-type fistula (type E) is usually made using nonionic water-soluble contrast or diluted barium during a radiographic study (Fig. 9). Demonstration of TEF with bronchoscopy can be helpful in diagnosis and operative planning (Fig. 10). The use of CT, virtual bronchoscopy, and MRI has also been reported, although their role in the diagnosis is not yet clear [12].

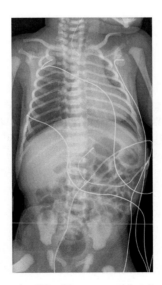

Fig. 7. Chest radiograph suggesting EA with a nasogastric tube curled in the proximal atretic pouch. (*Courtesy of* Polly Kochan, MD, Philadelphia, PA.)

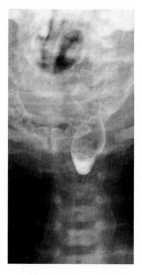

Fig. 8. Chest radiograph demonstrating the proximal atretic pouch outlined with dilute barium. (*Courtesy of* Polly Kochan, MD, Philadelphia, PA.)

The presence of components of the VACTERL association should increase suspicion for EA. Approximately 50% of patients who have EA or TEF present with additional birth defects. Complete evaluation should include: plain radiographs of the chest, abdomen, pelvis, and spine;

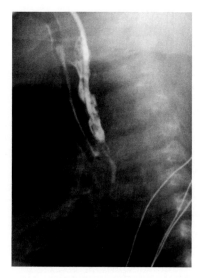

Fig. 9. Fluoroscopic image from a contrast esophagogram showing H-type (type E) fistula. (*Courtesy of* Polly Kochan, MD, Philadelphia, PA.)

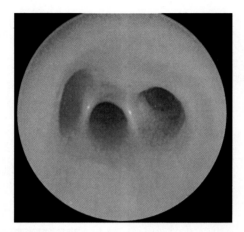

Fig. 10. Bronchoscopy demonstrating a distal tracheoesophageal fistula arising from the region of the carina in a patient who has EA with distal TEF (type C). (*Courtesy of* Glenn Isaacson, MD, Philadelphia, PA.)

ultrasound exams of the spine and kidneys; and echocardiography of the heart and aorta (Fig. 11).

Management

Preoperative

The main goal of preoperative management is to maintain the airway and to prevent lung damage from aspiration of gastric contents. This goal can be achieved by elevating the head of the bed and placing a suction catheter in the proximal pouch to prevent accumulation of saliva and mucus. Preoperative diagnostic studies should be performed expeditiously; echocardiographic evaluation of the heart and aorta are valuable in deciding the operative approach. The right chest is the preferred approach when a normal left-sided aortic arch is demonstrated.

Operative

Thoracotomy. The type of EA/TEF along with the length of the gap determines the timing and approach of the repair. The most common presentation, EA with distal TEF (type C), warrants an attempt at primary repair using the right-sided posterolateral extrapleural approach at the level of the fourth intercostal space (Fig. 12). The proximal pouch is mobilized in the cephalad direction to allow for approximation to the distal segment of the esophagus. The fistula is then carefully dissected to avoid damaging the trachea. The vagus nerve may be visualized as a landmark to identify the distal pouch as it enters the trachea; during this dissection care should be taken to avoid damage to its esophageal branches. The fistula is circumferentially mobilized and incised close to the trachea, leaving a rim of esophageal tissue on the trachea and

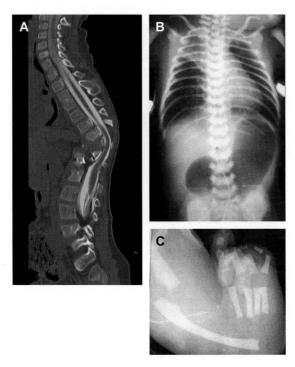

Fig. 11. (*A*) MRI of spine demonstrating vertebral anomalies in a neonate who has EA; (*B*) Plain radiograph demonstrating duodenal atresia in a neonate who has EA; (*C*) Plain radiograph showing limb anomalies (absence of radius and thumb). (*Courtesy of* Polly Kochan, MD, Philadelphia, PA.)

placing interrupted nonabsorbable sutures to close the fistula and support the resulting weakening in the trachea (Fig. 13). Dissection of the distal esophagus should be limited to avoid damaging its sparse blood supply. The anastomosis of the proximal esophageal pouch to the distal segment is usually achieved end-to-end using a set of two opposing traction sutures to achieve approximation of the two segments. The next step is placement of interrupted fine absorbable sutures through full thickness of the esophagus beginning at the posterior wall with the knots tied inside the lumen. An 8 French tube is passed down the esophagus with the end distal to the site of anastomosis, usually into the stomach, and interrupted sutures are placed in the anterior wall with extraluminal knots (Fig. 14). If the surgeon observes high anastomotic tension, the Haight two-layer telescoping anastomosis may achieve a better operative outcome. Another approach may be an end-to-side anastomosis or the performance of circular myotomies to gain needed esophageal length. Once the anastomosis is complete, a 10 or 12 French chest tube is usually placed in the area of the repair and secured to the chest wall. Some surgeons elect to place a transanastomotic feeding tube to encourage early enteral feeding. The chest wall is closed in layers with appropriate suture materials [2,3].

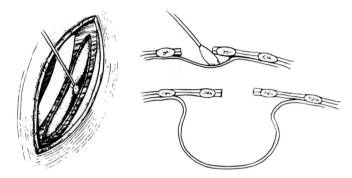

Fig. 12. Blunt dissection of the pleura away from the chest wall to create an extrapleural approach to the esophagus. (*From* Harmon CM, Coran AG. Congenital anomalies of the esophagus. In: Grosfeld JL, O'Neill Jr JA, Fonkalsrud EW, Coran AG, editors. Pediatric Surgery. 6th edition. Philadelphia: Mosby; 2006. p. 1059; with permission.)

Thoracoscopy. Advances in pediatric endoscopic surgery have resulted in the application of thoracoscopy to the management of EA. The first report of thoracoscopic repair was published in 1999 by Lobe and colleagues [13]. The advantages of using a minimally invasive approach include decreased

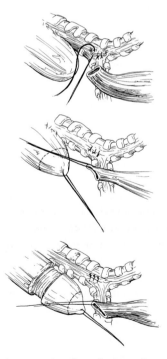

Fig. 13. Closure of TEF and preparation for primary end-to-end esophageal anastomosis. (*From* Harmon CM, Coran AG. Congenital anomalies of the esophagus. In: Grosfeld JL, O'Neill Jr JA, Fonkalsrud EW, Coran AG, editors. Pediatric Surgery. 6th edition. Philadelphia: Mosby; 2006. p. 1060; with permission.)

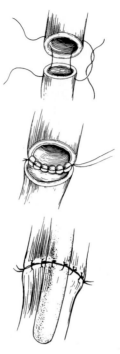

Fig. 14. Single-layer esophageal anastomosis. (*A*) Corner stitches are placed and the knots are tied on the outside. (*B*) The posterior row is placed with the knots tied on the inside. (*C*) The anterior row completes the anastomosis over a tube with the knots tied on the outside. (*From* Harmon CM, Coran AG. Congenital anomalies of the esophagus. In: Grosfeld JL, O'Neill Jr JA, Fonkalsrud EW, Coran AG, editors. Pediatric Surgery. 6th edition. Philadelphia: Mosby; 2006. p. 1060; with permission.)

morbidity associated with thoracotomy (respiratory compromise, postthoracotomy pain, postoperative recovery time, scoliosis, shoulder girdle weakness, chest wall asymmetry) and improved visualization with a magnifying camera. Disadvantages to performing the repair thoracoscopically include difficulty maneuvering instruments in the small working space and inability to place more than one suture at a time, causing increased tension and increased risk for suture material tearing through the tissue.

Prerequisites to a successful thoracoscopic repair include stable condition of the infant, a surgeon skilled in minimally invasive surgery, and adequate support from the anesthesia team. Absolute contraindications to endoscopic approach include severe hemodynamic instability, significant prematurity, or weight less than 1500 g. Relative contraindications include severe congenital cardiac defects, birth weight 1500 to 2000 g, or significant abdominal distention because of a proximal bowel atresia [14,15].

Operative management for thoracoscopic repair includes general anesthesia with endotracheal intubation, preferably of the left mainstem bronchus. The infant is placed in the prone position with the right side elevated to a 45° angle. Proper port placement is essential to obtain good visualization of the thoracic cavity and to allow for necessary instrument manipulation. The first 3- to 5-mm cannula is placed in the posterior axillary line at the level of fifth intercostal space, carbon dioxide is insufflated into the thoracic cavity, and a 30° camera is advanced through the port. One 5-mm port is placed in the midaxillary line one to two intercostal spaces above and one 3-mm port is placed in the midaxillary line one to two intercostal spaces below the laparoscope port; both are used for instruments, which should approximate at about a 90° angle. A fourth port is occasionally needed to achieve good lung retraction, although it is usually unnecessary. Once the fistula and the proximal pouch are identified, the surgeon should proceed with the dissection, division of the fistula, and anastomosis of the proximal and distal segments in the same basic steps as those described for thoracotomy [14,15].

Repair of long-gap atresia. Long-gap EA (usually type A) is defined as a gap of approximately 2.5 cm with the two segments not readily approximated without considerable tension. The traditional approach to the management of long-gap EA/TEF is to perform an initial feeding gastrostomy and to wait several weeks for spontaneous esophageal growth. Although performing the feeding gastrostomy, it is important to try to place the stoma closer to the lesser curvature to preserve the vascular supply of the greater curvature in case a reversed gastric tube is needed for esophageal replacement. Delayed primary repair may be accomplished once the segments are of sufficient length. Howard and Myers [16] pioneered the use of daily bougienage of the proximal pouch to encourage its growth. Placing bougies or contrast in proximal and distal pouches (through the gastrostomy) allows for the gap to be periodically measured with fluoroscopic imaging (Fig. 15). The application of an electromagnetic field to metal devices in the two respective pouches to promote growth and allow the gap to narrow has also been described [17], as has application of hydrostatic pressure to induce growth in the distal pouch [18]. Other techniques to elongate the esophageal segments included the use of proximal and distal circular myotomies and growth promotion using magnets, stringed beads, guide wires, and steel bars [17,19–21].

John Foker describes an innovative technique for assessment and repair of long-gap EA with or without TEF, which begins with dissection of the proximal and distal pouches and placement of four traction sutures on each segment without entering the lumen (Fig. 16). Primary repair is usually achievable if the segments are easily approximated, whereas if the surgeon perceives a significant amount of tension a multistaged operative approach may be necessary. Such an approach involves placing internal traction sutures from the upper and lower pouches under tension in the prevertebral fascia below and above the thoracotomy incision, respectively; in ultra long-gap these traction sutures are brought out through the intercostal

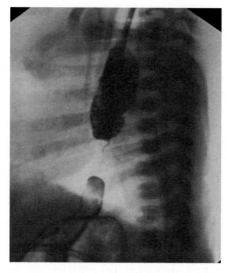

Fig. 15. Fluoroscopic image with contrast in the proximal pouch and distal pouch demonstrating the length of the gap in a type A EA (long gap variant).

spaces and tied over silastic buttons on the posterior chest wall (Fig. 17). Consequently, tension can be increased daily to promote rapid growth of the two segments. Clips may be placed on the ends of the two segments so that the advancement may be followed by plain film radiography. A second thoracotomy is then performed to achieve a primary end-to-end anastomosis. In Foker's series [22], adequate growth of the proximal and distal pouches occurred in 8 to 18 days to allow for primary repair.

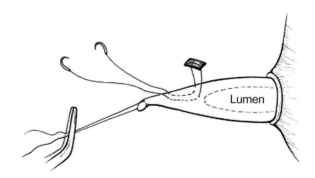

Fig. 16. Foker technique illustrating dissection of the distal pouch and placement of four pledgeted traction sutures on each segment without entering the lumen. (*From* Foker JE, Kendall T, Catton K, et al. A flexible approach to achieve a true primary repair for all infants with esophageal atresia. Semin Pediatr Surg 2005;14(1):8–15; with permission).

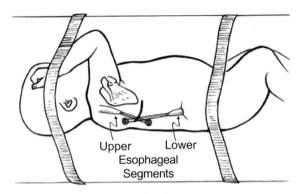

Fig. 17. Foker technique illustrating the traction sutures exiting the chest wall above and below the thoracotomy incision and tied over silastic buttons therefore allowing the tension to be increased daily. (*From* Foker JE, Kendall T, Catton K, et al. A flexible approach to achieve a true primary repair for all infants with esophageal atresia. Semin Pediatr Surg 2005;14(1):8–15; with permission).

Kimura and colleagues [23] developed a technique of multistaged extra-thoracic elongation of the proximal esophageal pouch that subsequently permits approximation and anastomosis of the two segments. Initial cervical approach involves freeing the proximal esophageal segment and creating an esophagostomy on the anterior chest wall through which "sham" oral infant feeding is administered and collected in an ostomy bag; nutrition is supplied by a gastrostomy tube until the repair is complete. Two months following the initial operation the esophagostomy is revised and placed lower on the chest wall. Once the proximal and distal pouches are approximated, a definitive end-to-end anastomosis is performed by way of a thoracotomy.

Although added complications of a multistage repair of long-gap atresia exist, the benefits of attaining repair of the native esophagus clearly decrease life-long morbidities for the patient. Complications of a multistaged repair include adhesions, anastomotic leaks, development of strictures (usually successfully managed using dilation), recurrence of fistulas, disorders of motility, and gastroesophageal reflux. Nevertheless, anastomosis of the native esophageal segments is a better option in the long term for patients who have long-gap atresia as compared with esophageal replacement [22,23].

Esophageal replacement. Esophageal replacement is necessary for patients in whom repair of the native esophagus is not feasible. Various techniques for replacement have been described using the stomach, small intestine, and colon. Gastric transposition to reestablish continuity of the upper gastrointestinal tract has been found to be effective in a large series of patients [24,25]. Another technique, first described by Schärli, uses the lesser curvature of the stomach to create a 3- to 4-cm tube for replacement of necessary esophageal length [26]. Similar techniques may be used to create a reversed or isoperistaltic gastric tube using the greater curvature of the stomach

[27,28]. Likewise, the uses of jejunal, ileal, or colonic segments for esophageal replacement have been described. Complications of these operations include dysmotility, dysphagia, difficulty feeding, gastroesophageal reflux, stricture, dilation of the nonnative segment, fistula formation, and compromised pulmonary function. Although the survival rate for these patients is good (~95%), associated morbidities often require additional procedures or operations [24–29].

H-type tracheoesophageal fistula. Diagnosis of congenital H-type tracheoesophageal fistula (type E) may be challenging. Common presenting symptoms suspicious for H-type tracheoesophageal fistula (type E) include cough and choking during feeding, recurrent pulmonary infections, and aerophagia. Anatomically, the fistula courses in an oblique fashion from the posterior aspect of the trachea to the more caudal anterior aspect of the esophagus. If H-type TEF is suspected, a contrast esophagogram is usually diagnostic (see Fig. 9). Bronchoscopy at the time of surgery, confirms the anatomic location of the fistula, which is important in operative planning and allows placement of a catheter in the fistula tract. Generally if the fistula is at the level of the second thoracic vertebra (T2) or higher (70% of H-type TEF), repair should proceed through a cervical incision, whereas fistulae below T2 require a thoracic approach. Thoracoscopic and endoscopic repairs have also been described [30,31].

For high fistulae, a right cervical incision is made and the fistula identified with the assistance of intraoperative bronchoscopic catheter placement. The fistula is then approached by dissection within the tracheoesophageal groove. The recurrent laryngeal nerve should be identified and preserved, the fistula is ligated and divided, and the esophageal and tracheal openings are closed using single-layer interrupted sutures. A local muscle flap may be transposed between the repaired trachea and esophagus. A nasogastric tube is placed to provide enteral nutrition and is usually removed around the fifth postoperative day. The success of operative treatment is documented by contrast esophagogram on about postoperative day five, after which oral feeds are resumed [32].

Postoperative

In an uncomplicated repair without anastomotic tension, prompt extubation is desirable if the cardiopulmonary status is stable. If excessive tension is noted, some surgeons prefer keeping the infant intubated and on neuromuscular blockade, with the neck in flexion. The head of the bed should be elevated to minimize the amount of gastroesophageal reflux. If a transanastomotic feeding tube has been placed, early enteral feeding may be instituted with return of gastrointestinal motility. If a feeding tube has not been placed, a contrast esophagogram should be performed around the fifth postoperative day and if no leak is noted oral feeds may be initiated and the retropleural drain removed. If the contrast esophagogram demonstrates a leak, or if saliva is noted in the draining retropleural fluid, feeding is delayed and drain output is recorded to monitor the progression of the leak. Most small leaks can be managed conservatively and resolve spontaneously without need for reoperation.

Outcomes

Immediate postoperative complications and long-term outcomes for repair of EA with distal TEF (type C) are tabulated (Table 4) [33–37].

Short term

Advances in techniques of repair of EA/TEF and neonatal intensive care have increased survival rates up to 95%. Survival is strongly correlated with birth weight and associated anomalies, especially congenital cardiac defects. Common complications during early postoperative period include: (1) strictures may be see in up to 50% of patients (although they may not all be symptomatic) (Fig. 18), most of which are successfully managed with dilation techniques; (2) anastomotic leaks in 5% to 15%, most of which resolve spontaneously; (3) recurrent tracheoesophageal fistulas in approximately 10%,

Table 4
Summary of complications in patients undergoing operative repairs of esophageal atresia with or without tracheoesophageal fistula

	Thoracotomy					Thoracoscopy
	Manning et al [33]	Spitz et al [34]	Randolph et al [35]	Engum et al [36]	Yanchar et al [37]	Holcomb et al [14]
Publication year	1986	1987	1989	1995	2001	2005
Total number of patients (% of patients who have type C-EA and TEF)	224 (85%)	148 (87%)	118 (100%)[a]	227 (78%)	90 (100%)	104 (99%)
Complications						
Anastomotic leaks	8.5%	21%	15%	16%	17%	8%
Anastomotic stricture	19%	18%	31%	35%	17%	4%
Anastomotic revision	—	3%	5%	0.9%	—	2%
Gastroesophageal reflux	38%	18% (life-threatening episodes)	38%	58%	46%	—
Fundoplication	29%	18%	15%	25%	32%	24%
Tracheomalacia	10%	—	4%	15%	—	—
Aortopexy or tracheostomy	5%	16%	—	6%	—	7%
Recurrent TEF	6%	12%	8%	3%	3%	2%

[a] Data analysis is on 26 primary repairs only.

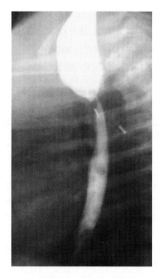

Fig. 18. Barium swallow showing an esophageal stricture at the site of esophageal anastomosis. (*Courtesy of* Polly Kochan, MD, Philadelphia, PA).

which may present with respiratory symptoms, such as cough and pneumonitis; (4) other respiratory problems in approximately 33% of patients [2,3,14,38–40].

Long term

Multiple investigators provide data on long-term complications of operative repair of EA/TEF. Most common sequelae in the first 5 years following repair include [41,42]:

Dysphagia (~45%)
Gastroesophageal reflux disease (~48%)
Respiratory infections (~29%)
Choking (~10%)
Esophageal stricture (20%–30%)
Symptomatic tracheomalacia (~15%)
Recurrent TEF (5%–10%)
Wheezing or bronchial hyperreactivity (~25%)
Chest wall deformities (~15%)

Health-related quality-of-life analysis revealed no significant differences in patients who had the repaired anomaly in comparison with healthy controls [43]. Although a significant increase in persistent respiratory symptoms was reported in patients who had EA/TEF, the incidence of severe respiratory symptoms was comparable to controls. Likewise, gastrointestinal symptoms, although persistent in approximately 10%, did not significantly affect quality of life in patients who had EA/TEF repairs in comparison with healthy controls [44].

Tracheomalacia is present in operative specimens in up to 75% of patients who have EA/TEF, although it is only clinically significant in about 10% to 20% of patients [42]. The defect is attributable to weakness of the cartilaginous rings of the trachea causing its anteroposterior collapse during the expiratory phase of the respiratory cycle. Symptoms are exaggerated with coughing, Valsalva maneuver, or any increase in intrathoracic pressure. In children who have EA/TEF repairs, the compression of the weakened trachea is exacerbated by the anterior-lying aorta and a posterior-lying dilated esophagus.

In tracheomalacia, the clinical presentation ranges from brassy or barking cough, stridor, dyspnea, recurrent pulmonary infections accompanied by wheezing, cyanosis, or frank apnea in most severe cases [2,3,43]. Diagnosis is made based on clinical history of EA/TEF and presenting symptoms and is confirmed by bronchoscopy, which demonstrates tracheal collapse during expiration (Fig. 19).

Mild to moderate symptoms of tracheomalacia are usually managed symptomatically, with operative measures reserved for severe cases causing life-threatening apneic episodes. The goal of operative treatment is to relieve pressure on the trachea. Historically, aortopexy was the treatment of choice in severe tracheomalacia, and involved the suturing of ascending aorta to the posterior surface of the sternum. Because the anterior aspect of the trachea adheres to the posterior aspect of the aorta, anterior compression of the tracheal lumen is relieved allowing it to remain patent during the entire respiratory cycle. The technique for aortopexy has been modified using various patches to prevent tension on the aorta. Recently, stenting technique has been suggested as a less invasive approach to the treatment of

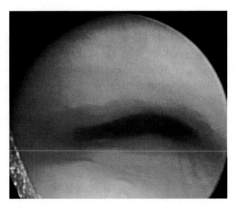

Fig. 19. Bronchoscopic image of tracheomalacia demonstrating tracheal collapse during expiration.

tracheomalacia [45]. Such stents have a high risk for delayed complications. In unremitting cases, tracheostomy allows for maturation and strengthening of the trachea [2,3,43].

Congenital esophageal stenosis

Congenital esophageal stenosis (CES) is a rare anomaly (1 in 25,000 to 50,000 live births) that is present at birth because of a malformation of the esophageal wall architecture [46,47] and is associated with other anomalies (gastrointestinal, cardiac, chromosomal) in up to one third of patients [47]. The incidence of CES is higher in Japan and is equal in males and females. Histologically, CES is classified into three groups:

Tracheobronchial remnants (cartilage, seromucous glands, and ciliated epithelium)
Fibromuscular thickening
Membranous webbing

Common presenting symptoms of CES are vomiting and dysphagia, especially with introduction of solid foods into the diet within the first year of life. Diagnosis is usually delayed but can be made by performing an esophagogram which may show an abrupt or tapered stenosis. Other diagnostic modalities include esophageal manometry, which may show an ectopic high-pressure segment above the lower esophageal sphincter; endoscopy, which may also be therapeutic; or 24-hour esophageal pH monitoring. Initial management is esophageal dilation using bougienage or a balloon catheter. Operative treatment is reserved for cases resistant to multiple dilations; this involves myotomy or resection of stenotic segment with primary anastomosis. Prognosis of CES patients is generally good, with most patients tolerating solid or semisolid foods [47,48].

Congenital esophageal duplication

Congenital esophageal duplication is a rare anomaly of the esophagus, with incidence of approximately 1 in 8000 live births, accounting for 10% to 15% of gastrointestinal duplications. The duplication results from aberrant vacuolization of the esophagus during the first trimester of gestation. It may be present in cystic or tubular form, although the cystic variant is much more common and usually lies in the posterior mediastinum. Histologic diagnostic criteria include [49]:

Attachment to the esophagus
Enclosure by two muscle layers
Lining by epithelium

Patients tend to present with respiratory symptoms, vomiting, regurgitation, and a possible neck mass. Although prenatal diagnosis has been

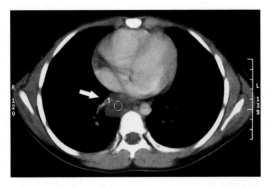

Fig. 20. CT scan of the thorax showing a cystic esophageal duplication.

reported [50], definitive diagnosis is usually made in early childhood using contrast esophagography. Transesophageal ultrasonography, endoscopy, CT scan (Fig. 20), and MRI may provide additional information on the precise location of the duplication. Because the duplication may increase in size with time and compress surrounding structures, operative resection is the treatment of choice. Depending on the size, location, and experience of the surgeon, posterolateral thoracotomy or thoracoscopy are the operative treatment options for the excision of an esophageal duplication (Fig. 21). Care must be taken in preserving the vagus and phrenic nerves, and the muscle and mucosal layers of the esophageal wall should be carefully reconstructed. Air insufflation by way of a nasogastric tube or flexible esophagoscopy should be used to assess the integrity of the esophagus

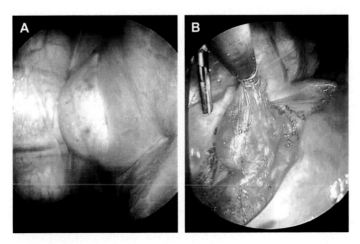

Fig. 21. (A) Thoracoscopic view of esophageal duplication. (B) Thoracoscopic resection of esophageal duplication.

following excision. Patient follow-up is necessary to assess for any complications, including leaks and changes in esophageal motility [51].

References

[1] Kluth D, Fiegel H. The embryology of the foregut. Semin Pediatr Surg 2003;12(1):3–9.

[2] Harmon CM, Coran AG, et al. Congenital anomalies of the esophagus. In: Grosfeld JL, O'Neill JA Jr, Fonkalsrud EW, editors. Pediatric surgery. 6th edition. Philadelphia: Mosby; 2006. p. 1051–81.

[3] Morrow S, Nakayama D, et al. Congenital malformations of the esophagus. In: Bluestone CD, Stool SE, Alper CM, editors. Pediatric otolaryngology. 4th edition. Philadelphia: WB Saunders; 2002. p. 1281–8.

[4] Bae JO, Widmann WD, Hardy MA. Cameron Haight: pioneer in the treatment of esophageal atresia. Curr Surg 2005;62(3):327–9.

[5] Waterston DJ, Carter RE, Aberdeen E. Oesophageal atresia: tracheo-oesophageal fistula. A study of survival in 218 infants. Lancet 1962;1:819–22.

[6] Spitz L, Kiely EM, Morecroft JA, et al. Oesophageal atresia: at risk groups for the 1990s. J Pediatr Surg 1994;29(6):723–5.

[7] Driver CP, Shankar KR, Jones MO, et al. Phenotypic presentation and outcome of esophageal atresia in the era of the Spitz classification. J Pediatr Surg 2001;36(9):1419–21.

[8] Beasley SW, Williams AK, Qi BQ, et al. The development of the proximal oesophageal pouch in the Adriamycin rat model of oesophageal atresia with tracheo-oesophageal fistula. Pediatr Surg Int 2004;20:548–50.

[9] Thompson DJ, Molello JA, Strebing RJ, et al. Teratogenicity of Adriamycin and daunomycin in the rat and rabbit. Teratology 1978;17(2):151–7.

[10] Felix JF, Keijzer R, van Dooren MF, et al. Genetics and developmental biology of oesophageal atresia and tracheo-oesophageal fistula: lessons form mice relevant for paediatric surgeons. Pediatr Surg Int 2004;20(10):731–6.

[11] Has R, Gunay S, Topuz S. Pouch sign in prenatal diagnosis of esophageal atresia. Ultrasound Obstet Gynecol 2004;23(5):523–4.

[12] Berrocal T, Madrid C, Novo S, et al. Congenital anomalies of the tracheobronchial tree, lung, and mediastinum: embryology, radiology, and pathology. Radiographics 2004;24(1): e17.

[13] Lobe TE, Rothenberg SS, Waldschmidt J, et al. Thoracoscopic repair of esophageal atresia in an infant: a surgical first. Pediatric Endosurgery and Innovative Techniques 1999;3:141–8.

[14] Holcomb GW, Rothenberg SS, Bax KM, et al. Thoracoscopic repair of esophageal atresia and tracheoesophageal fistula: a multi-institutional analysis. Ann Surg 2005;242(3):422–30.

[15] Rothenberg SS. Thoracoscopic repair of esophageal atresia and tracheo-esophageal fistula. Semin Pediatr Surg 2005;14(1):2–7.

[16] Howard R, Myers N. Esophageal atresia: a technique for elongating the upper pouch. Surgery 1965;58:725–9.

[17] Hendren WH, Hale JR. Esophageal atresia treated by electromagnetic bougienage and subsequent repair. J Pediatr Surg 1976;11(5):713–22.

[18] Vogel AM, Yang EY, Fishman SJ. Hydrostatic stretch-induced growth facilitating primary anastomosis in long-gap esophageal atresia. J Pediatr Surg 2006;41(6):1170–2.

[19] Livaditis A, Radberg L, Odensjo G. Esophageal end-to-end anastomosis: reduction of anastomotic tension by circular myotomy. Scand J Thorac Cardiovasc Surg 1972;6(2):206–14.

[20] Rehbein F, Schweder N. Reconstruction of the esophagus without colon transplantation in cases of atresia. J Pediatr Surg 1971;6(6):746–52.

[21] Gauderer MW. Delayed blind-pouch apposition, guide wire placement, and nonoperative establishment of luminal continuity in a child with long gap esophageal atresia. J Pediatr Surg 2003;38(6):906–9.

[22] Foker JE, Kendall T, Catton K, et al. A flexible approach to achieve a true primary repair for all infants with esophageal atresia. Semin Pediatr Surg 2005;14(1):8–15.

[23] Kimura K, Nishijima E, Tsugawa C, et al. Multistaged extrathoracic esophageal elongation procedure for long gap esophageal atresia: experience with 12 patients. J Pediatr Surg 2001; 36(11):1725–7.

[24] Spitz L, Keily E, Pierro A. Gastric transposition in children—a 21-year experience. J Pediatr Surg 2004;39(3):276–81.

[25] Hirschl RB, Yardeni D, Oldham K, et al. Gastric transposition for esophageal replacement in children: experience with 41 consecutive cases with special emphasis on esophageal atresia. Ann Surg 2002;236(4):531–41.

[26] Fernandez MS, Gutiérrez C, Ibáñez V, et al. Long-gap esophageal atresia: reconstruction preserving all portions of the esophagus by Schärli's technique. Pediatr Surg Int 1998; 14(1–2):17–20.

[27] McCollum MO, Rangel SJ, Blair GK, et al. Primary reversed gastric tube reconstruction in long gap esophageal atresia. J Pediatr Surg 2003;38(6):957–62.

[28] Borgnon J, Tounian P, Auber F, et al. Esophageal replacement by an isoperistaltic gastric tube: a 12 year experience. Pediatr Surg Int 2004;20:829–33.

[29] Séguier-Lipszyc E, Bonnard A, Aizenfisz S, et al. The management of long gap esophageal atresia. J Pediatr Surg 2005;40(10):1542–6.

[30] Allal H, Montes-Tapia F, Andina G, et al. Thoracoscopic repair of H-type tracheoesophageal fistula in the newborn: a technical case report. J Pediatr Surg 2004;39(10):1568–70.

[31] Tzifa KT, Maxwell EL, Chait P, et al. Endoscopic treatment of congenital H-type and recurrent tracheoesophageal fistula with electrocautery and histoacryl glue. Int J Pediatr Otorhinolaryngol 2006;70(5):925–30.

[32] Karnak I, Şenocak ME, Hiçsönmez A, et al. The diagnosis and treatment of H-type tracheoesophageal fistula. J Pediatr Surg 1997;32(12):1670–4.

[33] Manning PB, Morgan RA, Coran AG, et al. Fifty years' experience with esophageal atresia and tracheoesophageal fistula. Beginning with Cameron Haight's first operation in 1935. Ann Surg 1986;204(4):446–51.

[34] Spitz L, Kiely E, Brereton RJ. Esophageal atresia: five-year experience with 148 cases. J Pediatr Surg 1987;22(2):103–8.

[35] Randolph JG, Newman KD, Anderson KD. Current results in repair of esophageal atresia with tracheoesophageal fistula using physiologic status as a guide to therapy. Ann Surg 1989; 209(5):526–31.

[36] Engum SA, Grosfeld JL, West KA, et al. Analysis of morbidity and mortality in 227 cases of esophageal atresia and/or tracheoesophageal fistula over two decades. Arch Surg 1995; 130(5):502–9.

[37] Yanchar NL, Gordon R, Cooper M, et al. Significance of the clinical course and early upper gastrointestinal studies in predicting complications associated with repair of esophageal atresia. J Pediatr Surg 2001;36(5):815–22.

[38] Naik-Mathuria B, Olutoye OO. Foregut abnormalities. Surg Clin North Am 2006;86(2): 261–84.

[39] Tsai JY, Berkery L, Wesson DE, et al. Esophageal atresia and tracheoesophageal fistula: surgical experience over two decades. Ann Thorac Surg 1997;64(3):778–84.

[40] Deurloo JA, Smit BJ, Ekkelkamp S, et al. Oesophageal atresia in premature infants: an analysis of morbidity and mortality over a period of 20 years. Acta Paediatr 2004;93(3): 394–9.

[41] Little DC, Rescorla FJ, Grosfeld JLL, et al. Long-term analysis of children with esophageal atresia and tracheoesophageal fistula. J Pediatr Surg 2003;38(6):852–6.

[42] Kovesi T, Rubin S. Long-term complications of congenital esophageal atresia and/or tracheoesophageal fistula. Chest 2004;126(3):915–25.

[43] Deurloo JA, Ekkelkamp S, Hartman EE, et al. Quality of life in adult survivors of correction of esophageal atresia. Arch Surg 2005;140(10):976–80.

[44] Koivusalo A, Pakarinen MP, Turunen P, et al. Health-related quality of life in adult patients with esophageal atresia—a questionnaire study. J Pediatr Surg 2005;40(2):307–12.

[45] Filler RM, Forte V, Fraga JC, et al. The use of expandable metallic airway stents for tracheobronchial obstruction in children. J Pediatr Surg 1995;30(7):1050–5.

[46] Nishina T, Tsuchida Y, Saito S. Congenital esophageal stenosis due to tracheobronchial remnants and its associated anomalies. J Pediatr Surg 1981;16(2):190–3.

[47] Amae S, Nio M, Kamiyama T, et al. Clinical characteristics and management of congenital esophageal stenosis: a report on 14 cases. J Pediatr Surg 2003;38(4):565–70.

[48] Kawahara H, Oue T, Okuyama H, et al. Esophageal motor function in congenital esophageal stenosis. J Pediatr Surg 2003;38(12):1716–9.

[49] Wootton-Gorges SL, Eckel GM, Poulos ND, et al. Duplication of the cervical esophagus: a case report and review of literature. Pediatr Radiol 2002;32(7):533–5.

[50] Gul A, Tekoglu G, Aslan H, et al. Prenatal sonographic features of esophageal and ileal duplications at 18 weeks of gestation. Prenat Diagn 2004;24(12):969–71.

[51] Cioffi U, Bonavina L, De Simone M, et al. Presentation and surgical management of bronchogenic and esophageal duplication cysts in adults. Chest 1998;113(6):1492–6.

ELSEVIER
SAUNDERS

Otolaryngol Clin N Am
40 (2007) 245–249

OTOLARYNGOLOGIC
CLINICS
OF NORTH AMERICA

Index

Note: Page numbers of article titles are in **boldface** type.

0030-6665/07/$ - see front matter © 2007 Elsevier Inc. All rights reserved.
doi:10.1016/S0030-6665(07)00010-2

oto.theclinics.com

Moving?

Make sure your subscription moves with you!

To notify us of your new address, find your **Clinics Account Number** (located on your mailing label above your name), and contact customer service at:

E-mail: elspcs@elsevier.com

800-654-2452 (subscribers in the U.S. & Canada)
407-345-4000 (subscribers outside of the U.S. & Canada)

Fax number: 407-363-9661

Elsevier Periodicals Customer Service
6277 Sea Harbor Drive
Orlando, FL 32887-4800

*To ensure uninterrupted delivery of your subscription, please notify us at least 4 weeks in advance of move.